CW00552806

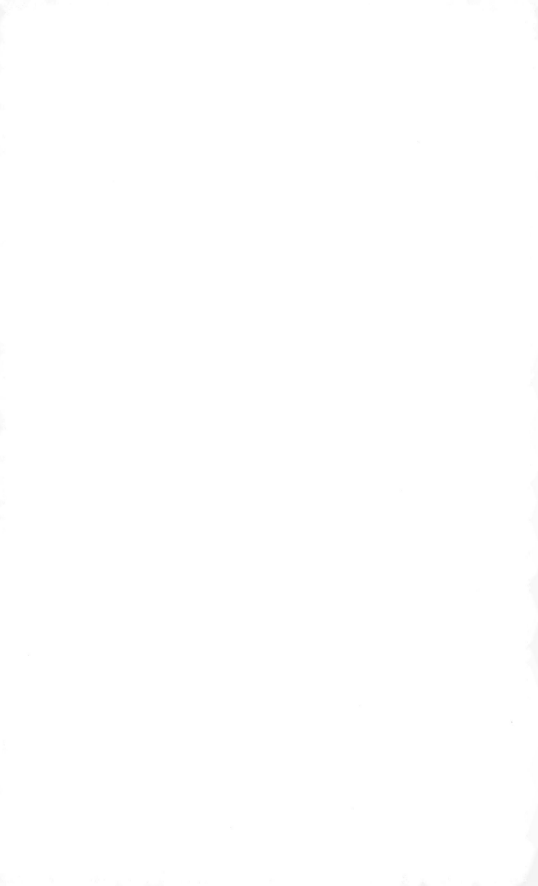

A New Health Era

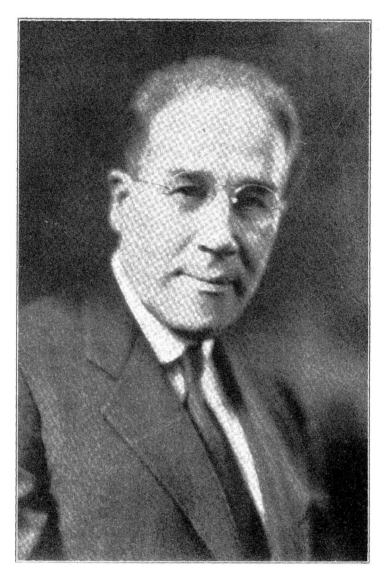

WILLIAM HOWARD HAY, M.D.

A New Health Era

By

WILLIAM HOWARD HAY M.D.

Medical Director
HAY SYSTEM Inc.

Sanatorium Hotel Headquarters
BRIARCLIFF LODGE
BRIARCLIFF MANOR N.Y.

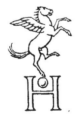

GEORGE G. HARRAP & CO. LTD.
LONDON   BOMBAY   SYDNEY

Dedication

THIS small volume is not dedicated to any one individual, even though many have contributed materially to the subject matter through example and recorded experience.

No, it is dedicated to man himself, the downtrodden and much exploited genus homo, who in matters of his own health and efficiency has ever been the goat.

Benjamin Franklin said long ago that but one per cent of humanity is capable of independent thought and correct reasoning.

Maybe he is right, so perhaps this volume will be read profitably by but this small percentage of the genus, though it is hoped that the other ninety-nine per cent may find here something to stimulate thought of the independent variety, and perhaps correct reasoning also.

It is with the hope that a somewhat more cheerful outlook on health and continued life may be stimulated in those less than well that this volume is dedicated to the victim himself.

TABLE OF CONTENTS

Introduction

EVER since the recent World War there has appeared a tendency to analyze, to inspect, to take with a grain of salt every new doctrine offered, and not many of the old and accepted doctrines have escaped this same apparent tendency.

It takes some great cataclysm such as the recent war to jar us out of many beliefs that have been accepted for ages simply because we were too lazy to properly analyze them.

The world has begun to awaken, to scan critically, to see independently, to reason correctly; and when we can think there is still hope for us.

Scientists who have achieved much, who have proved to the world their ability to think independently and reason correctly, are still unable to apply these mental traits to their own bodily condition. They seem to have such respect for the thoughts of others outside their own field of research, that they go to the clinic and in all good faith accept the findings of a group of men who have made a deep study of disease, perhaps, yet who are finite minds, subject to all the mistakes in observation and reasoning from cause to effect that is usual in every other field of endeavor.

If we knew the intimate body processes we might perhaps call medicine a science; but the internal chemistry and zymotic activity of the body are still a very deep secret, as enzymes, or ferments, are not subject to exact chemical analysis, and their processes must be guessed at, largely.

The writer has practiced medicine and general surgery for well over forty years. For the first sixteen years of this time he was called orthodox, accepting the statements of so-called authorities as final wisdom, as he was taught to do, both in arts and sciences college and later during his whole medical training.

It was while studying medicine that his private quiz master suggested that he not confine his study to the authors suggested or prescribed by his teachers at the university, but read several authors; it was then that it began to dawn on him that there was little agreement among these various authors, even on those subjects that were at that time supposed to be well-grounded in science.

He studied those authors prescribed in order to pass a creditable examination on the subjects discussed by these men, but his answers were always given with a certain degree of reservation, remembering divergent opinions of other authors, and he soon came to hold a sort of open mind on all questions generally accepted as settled.

During these forty-two years since graduation he has not failed to note this very same condition among authors, scarce any two agreeing on most phases of every subject.

Now, if medicine is not sure, why should the layman not feel all at sea in regard to his own condition?

This same layman will go to his physician and with the most implicit and child-like faith take everything this man says as law and gospel; or he used to do this far more universally before this awakening already alluded to.

When doctors cannot agree, does it not seem that there is something radically wrong with the whole conception of disease?

One specialist whom I have known for many years treats asthma, yet he is a fearful wheezer himself.

Another specializes in rheumatism and arthritis, but he is a sufferer from the very same malady he treats; also his wife suffers equally from the same condition.

Still another specializes in digestive troubles, while both he and the members of his family are victims of various digestive disorders.

Verily, it looks like the blind leading the blind.

Someone has not been thinking or this state of affairs could not exist; or is disease such a misunderstood thing that even those who make a life study of it are to be excused for not understanding it?

The writer practiced according to the light of the best thought of his time, supposedly, for sixteen years, feeling all the time that his own mistakes in diagnosis, prognosis and treatment were not any more glaring than those of his neighbors. And as his respect for authority had early suffered through study of many instead of few authors, it is not surprising that he developed a sort of fatalism in treating his cases, feeling that those who were to die did so according to program, and those who were elected to live were gladly accepted as stars in his medical crown, just as we all do.

If the patient recovers, great is the glory of medicine, but if he dies, it is just too bad, or the Lord took him away from a sinful world, and probably from a fate still worse; and we are at least comforted by the feeling that science had done all it could.

After sixteen years of busy practice, devoted largely to general surgery, he broke down; proving that he knew as little as the rest, of the predisposing causes of disease.

Bright's disease developed, with high blood pressure, and finally dilated heart, a condition for which there is no relief in medicine, or at least but temporary relief, and he was forced to consider himself on the shelf, or very near it.

But during the long nights of wakefulness and labored breathing his mental processes seemed to be very much alive, and he actually thought, yes, dared to think fundamentally, forgetting the opiates with which he had formerly excused himself for following the crowd, and he reached certain conclusions that were worth application as a frank experiment.

He began to eat fundamentally; to take only such things as he believed were intended by nature as foods for man, taking these in their natural form, and in quantities no greater than seemed to be necessary for present need.

His troubles slipped away, till at the end of three months he was again able to run long distances without distress. His weight decreased from 225 lbs. to 175 lbs.; years seemed to fall away from him, and he felt younger and stronger than before for many years.

This experience further deepened his conviction that there must be something about disease that we had not understood, for here was his own case recovering from a condition that the best authorities said was incurable. To prove that he was definitely and permanently cured he has since that time taken out life insurance to the amount of more than one hundred and fifty thousand dollars, without any rating-up or lessening of the amount of insurance asked for.

All this happened nearly twenty-six years ago, and the same high level of health persists today as after full recovery from this supposedly incurable disease.

Following this experience, four years were devoted to treatment of disease along dietary lines in an effort to prove or disprove that the body is merely a composite of what goes into it daily in the form of food and drink; and the four years furnished proof in plenty that, given the right food in the right way, anybody can be as well as desired.

Not only so, but since this theory was definitely accepted as a fact, thousands of cases of every sort, the majority suffering from some form of so-called incurable disease, have passed through the same form of treatment, as is necessary to create the body of right materials. While many of these were too far degenerated to recover, yet the history of the entire treatment period showed attempted regeneration on the part of the body in every case, and only those who were either too far gone, or who did not continue to follow the plan of regenerative eating prescribed, failed to recover completely.

So the writer has been definitely forced to believe that if

the body is nourished correctly it cannot develop disease; and even if disease is gone far the body will recover, unless there has been too great destruction of some vital organ or organs.

But three things are necessary for recovery before this point of organic destruction is reached: first, a desire to recover; not a weak wish to be better, but a burning desire that is willing to sacrifice much, to go through hell, if need be, to recover; second, a knowledge of the modus or method by which this return to health may be made; and third, the will power, the determination, the guts, to see the thing through. Equipped with these three requisites to recovery, nothing can interfere with this, only supposing that no vital organ is hopelessly degenerated.

These requisites do not comprehend a clinic, a medicine, or an operating room; for recovery rests with the individual, the one chiefly interested.

The writer has in mind many cases of supposedly incurable disease that have recovered completely; so completely that their health is now at the highest point it has ever attained, even in childhood, and who are continually regenerating; doing things this year that they were not able to do last year; developing endurance and efficiency with each year, and enjoying life as never before.

These are not the exception but the usual rule; where the food intake is properly managed continually; for the other adjuvants to a high state of health will usually follow an improved nutritional state, and one will voluntarily take exercise, sun, air, bathing, deep breathing, none of which will be of much service in recovering health without the fundamental one of correct nutrition.

Therefore, this unpretentious attempt to point out the way of regeneration to all the degenerating mass outside this knowledge at present, is to be excused, and in no sense accepted as merely another attempt to break into print.

The writer wishes to assure every reader that the full proof

[15]

of the position taken in regard to nutrition is open to individual test at the hands of every reader, and he hereby assures such that merely separating into compatible groups the foods ordinarily eaten will bring such results as will insure the reader's full acceptance of the whole theory here set forth.

After all, are not our bodies in the veriest sense merely a composite of what we eat and drink daily, yearly, as a life habit? If we doubt this, then of what is the body built and rebuilt daily?

If we accept the statement above, then we are under the necessity of admitting that it does make a vital difference, it does seem important to our health, that the foods used should represent those needed by the body at the time, and the chemistry of digestion surely does become of vital importance in our consideration of what we eat and how we eat it.

If your doctor tells you to eat plenty of good nourishing food in order to keep well and strong, change doctors, for such a man has missed in his training the fundamentals of nutrition. Any man who says it does not make any difference what we eat or how we combine the foods used should be forever debarred from giving any advice to the sick or those who do not wish to become sick in the future.

In all considerations of health or illness, the manner and the matter of food rank so much higher than all others that this work is to be confined largely to discussion of food and its relation to health, happiness, efficiency and long life; not forgetting that there are many other considerations that are important, but believing that if correct eating habits prevail the rest will take care of themselves.

CHAPTER I.

History of Medicine

FROM the beginning of recorded time man has looked to physicians of some sort for the healing of his many afflictions; and always he has seemed to be kept in ignorance of his own part, his own responsibilities, in the matter of health or disease.

It seems strange, yet it is true, that everyone seems to feel qualified to prescribe for the illnesses of his friends and acquaintances, yet very much in the dark about his own afflictions.

Let your friends know that you have a common cold and they are prolific with directions for its proper treatment, even though they themselves may be suffering from the same affliction at the very time.

Lay prescribing is not only common, it is well-nigh universal.

Medicine did not originate with Hippocrates, the so-called father of medicine, by any means, though he is generally credited with the first attempt to set out in order what seemed to be a scientific observation of disease in its various phases, and a system of treatment that seemed the best course then extant.

Medicine was always practiced in some form, as each sufferer was led to apply for help to someone else, someone whom he believed to know more about what to do than he himself did.

This tendency gradually led to the setting aside of a class whose business it was to attend to the ills of the tribe or community; physicians, in other words.

Superstition and fear have always ruled the consideration of disease from the standpoint of the sufferer himself. Fear has been the means of exploitation always, and still is today, after all the years of failure to reach a scientific basis for the consideration of either disease or its management.

We exploit those who do not know as much as we think we know, which is merely human nature applied selfishly.

So this superstitious attitude that has always handicapped the ill has lent this class to continual exploitation, even as today; for if the surgeon cannot raise fear in the mind of the victim, he is not hugely successful in securing consent for an operation which the patient himself fears but little less than the condition that he does not understand, which has led him to consult the surgeon.

As wisdom has increased, so has sorrow, just as Solomon said; for while we have learned to understand much that was formerly unknown to us, yet at the same time the increased knowledge is too often used to add fright to our internal troubles, and we are too often frightened into operations, most of which never should have occurred.

Charms, incantations, exorcisms of supposedly unfriendly and harmful spirits, all these were the form of treatment followed before man became wise enough to understand that spirits had nothing to do with our maladies. But I am wondering if these ancient misunderstandings are not closely related to our present fear of germs.

As the anatomy of the body became better understood, the way was opened for the surgeon, who sought to rearrange the internal works to his satisfaction, and with the hope that this would in some way improve conditions.

Barbers and priests reigned during the dark ages, the barber being the surgeon, because he knew how to cut, presumably, the priest was the one who corresponded to the present day internist; his intercessions being supposed to placate those spirits that could be reached in this way, or to exorcise those too unfriendly to listen to his intercession.

And man, the goat, always paid for these ministrations, for they could not be performed for nothing.

[18]

This tendency of man in illness to look to someone else who was supposed to know some means of vicarious relief from the ills from which he suffers, has always been the motive for service along the lines of treatment for disease, and still continues to be the prime motive for this whole system of treatment, not more so in the dark ages than today.

This tendency has come from man's misunderstanding of his own body and its processes, a misunderstanding that has furnished opportunity for exploitation in all times. Even as in the so-called dark ages, today the case is no different, and man himself creates this seeming need for expert guidance in matters of health and disease.

It has been discovered that thousands of years ago in Egypt surgery had reached a certain degree of efficiency that permitted of internal operations, trephining of the skull, section of the abdomen, and much that we today practice, that we thought originated with the present civilization. Also, the administration of drug remedies had been practiced long before our present civilization was in existence, showing that even so long ago there was some sort of medical training, and some form of recognized treatment for disease.

Galen brought us a fair understanding of anatomy, and his work, combined with that of Hippocrates, was the foundation of our present system of medical and surgical treatment.

This all presupposes an extraneous cause for disease, a false conception of the very nature of the thing, for disease is intrinsic to the body, created by the body itself, through manufacture of the acid end-products of digestion and metabolism, ashes of the body itself and the oxidative processes by which it maintains its activities.

When these ashes or end-products are manufactured in amount greater than can be fully eliminated, we suffer from retention of these, and a state develops that is variously called auto-intoxication, acid-autotoxicosis, toxaemia, self-poisoning, or whatever you wish to call it, expressing this manufacture and retention of these irritating acid end-products.

The science of medicine takes no cognizance of this accumulation till disease, that is, till definite pathology has developed, and then the condition is submitted to the most intimate study. This is merely locking the stable door after the horse has been stolen, a rather feeble gesture, not in any sense constructive treatment.

Yet this is the only sort of treatment considered orthodox by the medical profession, and, whether the answer is medical or surgical, it must be evident to anyone who can reason that such treatment has little value, for it is dealing with effects, not in any sense with causes.

Medicine has grown into a major so-called science, and only because humanity has continued to build up this increasingly toxic state that furnishes continually much clinical material.

So medicine is really a creation of a class set aside for treatment of human ills, not for prevention of these, (and medicine begins just where individual care ceases) for the purpose of patching the machine that has been ruined by the mistreatment of the average human, either from misunderstanding of body needs or from a carelessness as to the results.

We need not blame medicine for this condition, as the cause is individual, chargeable to the victim himself.

Thus medicine has flourished in all times from the ignorance and inattention of the individual in matters of his own health and efficiency; and the continued need for repairing the damage we do to our bodies will persist till we learn to accept our individual responsibilities in the matter of keeping ourselves as well as we should and as well as we can be, if we understand better the self-created causes of our many ills.

As the medical fraternity has increased in numbers, so also has their training become more and more involved and diversified, till now to be a doctor of medicine requires eight years of preparation, after leaving the high school. This means two years of pre-medical work, four years of direct medical study, and two years of resident work as interne in a recognized hospital.

If one is going into surgery there is usually added to this a year or more of study in prominent surgical clinics; and if one of the specialties is contemplated there is one or more years of this special study necessary before going into practice.

With this large expenditure of time and money, it is not at all strange that the recent graduate, who is now a potential doctor of medicine, feels a great need of some return on his capital invested, nor is it to be wondered at that every case presented for treatment is looked on as grist for his mill. If such patient can escape without some expensive line of treatment, or some lucrative major operation, he is to be congratulated.

Dr. Roger Morris, of Detroit, Mich., says that when he sends his patient to the group clinic he expects him to return with diagnosis of as many different diseases as are represented by the clinic as a whole. If he returns without a diagnosis of heart disease in some form, he knows well that the heart specialist was not in.

This is the natural tendency, for each sees the thing he most wishes to see in the patient, finds the thing he has been taught to find, and unless the physician is a super-human this is to be wholly expected.

One prominent nose and throat surgeon admitted to the writer that tonsils do recover without their removal; yet this same man made the statement the same evening before his medical group that if he were persuaded that tonsils could be corrected without their removal he would forego all of his tonsillectomies.

The reaction on his medical brethren was a big "horse laugh," for they remembered that this same man gets five hundred dollars for each removal of the tonsils, and they were sure he was human and could not resist this large fee. Nor could he, for he was human, and he does remove tonsils wholesale, just as before he made this statement to the writer, just between us two, that the tonsils do recover without their removal.

Dr. Charles Mayo said a few years ago that nine-tenths of the internal surgical operations of today never should have been done. He is far too conservative in that statement, for it is the writer's firm conviction that ninety-nine percent of all internal operations performed today never should have been done, and the other one per cent should be done by some sure-enough surgeon who has proved that he is qualified to open the body cavities without doing irreparable harm.

Today anyone having the letters "M.D." after his name is legally empowered to cut into anyone who will stand for it, whether or not he has ever before performed the kind of operation he is about to perform. If his patient dies it is surely too bad, but there is nothing to do about it, for the patient's consent absolves him from all blame, even if he used undue means to create in his patient a fear of the condition that negatived his fear of the operation.

How all this danger could be so easily obviated, if each one understood his own equipment better, and knew why he is less than well and just what to do to return to better conditions!

Fear resulting from ignorance of the body processes is the occasion for the creation of this class of physicians and surgeons and this same fear perpetuates them.

Learn the true nature of disease and how to keep the body at the normal continually, and you can laugh at the physician and surgeon, for you will then not need their ministrations.

Medicine has ever been considered an honorable calling, and the profession is an honorable one, surely, but physicians and surgeons are merely humans especially trained to do certain things, and being human, are subject to all the errors of judgment of any human being. When we add to this the fact that they are dealing largely with imponderable quantities, it is not difficult to see that errors that may cause loss of life can easily creep into their considerations of disease.

When humanity becomes wise enough to understand the origin of its own illnesses and sane enough to correct these causes, then the physician will gradually become the teacher and watch-dog of health, not the tinkerer with the end-results of the many mistakes now committed daily against health by the average man or woman in every walk of life in every civilized country on the globe.

That such a time will come there is no doubt, but that it will be within the life of the present generation is extremely doubtful.

It is human nature to shrink from too close self-examination when habit is under consideration; and it is not human nature to assume any disagreeable responsibility, when a convenient belief persists that no matter how we behave personally, there always can be some vicarious substitute for self-government, with its painful necessity for thought.

The word "doctor" means teacher, and a teacher he should be, not a tinkerer.

The writer seems to have grown up with the thought of medicine as a calling, for he is unable to remember when he considered any other vocation; yet had he known the futility of medical practice he could never have been persuaded to go through the painful years of preparation necessary for the work.

He went to New York with the deep conviction that if one were smart enough he could devise means for the control of all disease; but in three short years this idea was thoroughly dispelled, and he left the city knowing that even the smartest brains in medicine were sure of very little in the treatment of disease.

It is not strange that a cult has grown up that can flourish

[23]

on nothing less than the infirmities and calamities of their fellow men; for so long as these illnesses persist, just so long will there be occasion for the practice of medicine.

It is an honorable thing, a splendid thing, to relieve the sufferings and illnesses of one's fellows, but it is a far better thing to prevent these same sufferings, though it can be done in no other way than by the individual himself.

The vast majority of people would live so as to prevent illnesses if they could be made to believe that these are preventable, by means of a few very simple changes in the ordinary dietary habit. One who would not be willing to do this, knowing that he could in this way prevent all illness, would not be worth the instruction necessary to save him from ill health and suffering. Such would be a deliberate suicide.

Throughout the entire history of medicine you will find that all energy and all teaching is directed against disease after it is developed; and only in the past few years has any great amount of attention been directed toward the beginnings of disease.

It is an evidence of progress when we have a national board that we call Public Health; and the Public Health Service, P. H. S., is becoming a real factor nationally, though still confining too much of its attention to serum treatment, under the guise of prevention, even though it has not been proved, and cannot be proved, that these means prevent anything.

If the P. H. S. will devote itself to perfecting drainage, sewering, the safeguarding of foods sold to the public, the guarding of all foods and drinks against contamination, adulteration, and harmful preservatives, they will abundantly fulfil the mission their founders had in mind; but when they invade the field of serumology they begin to lose their usefulness.

Medicine may be an art, distantly related to the ancient black art, but still art of a kind, but—a science? Never, till we know far more of the body and its intimate processes than we now know.

To fulfil the ideal mission of medicine it should be placed on a wholly altruistic basis, so that no thought of individual gain or personal prestige could possibly enter into our consideration of the healing art or profession.

This will undoubtedly require governmental supervision, with governmental appointment and continual control; a condition not likely to develop in our time, perhaps never in a government that is supposed to grant the utmost freedom to its citizens in earning their living.

If the victim of unnecessary and inefficient surgery were to become a menace to the liberty of the unsuccessful surgeon, if every unnecessary and bunglesome operation were to be immediately punished by fine, imprisonment, or revocation of license, there would be but little surgery to swell the business of the mortician; but so long as the medical profession is organized and protected against suits for malpractice, it will still be impossible to bring these unfortunate surgical deaths into the same class with those injured or killed by their employer's negligence.

Manufacturers are continually forced to contest damage suits resulting from injuries to their employees; even the pedestrian who thumbs a ride in your car is a potential damage suit if injured while your passenger. But the surgeon may attempt an operation that is unnecessary, that he knows to be unnecessary, and without the conscious skill to carry through successfully the thing undertaken, yet he is immune to suit or prosecution, because the law presumes that the doctor can do no wrong; that being thoroughly educated in the body, and licensed by the state to earn his living through medicine or surgery, therefore he has fulfilled all that is required of him, and accidents happening under his administration of illness are in some mysterious manner outside of or above the law.

Unless there is some sort of check on the activities of the ambitious and money-hungry surgeons, we are in danger of developing a race sans appendices, sans gall bladders, sans tonsils, sans everything in the way of appurtenances that can be spared without taking the life of the subject.

Because surgery has developed a skill and technique that allows of a certain degree of safety from death, does not argue that for this reason the operator is justified in performing operations that mutilate the subject; and most operations not only do not improve the condition of the victim, but in many respects cripple him for life.

It has been the writer's opportunity to see many thousands of surgical cripples, those who have lost organs and who never again will be as well as before their cherished operations, yet it is fairly safe to bet that in the vast majority of cases each victim believes that his operation saved his life at the time.

If these same victims were to know the actual truth, that without the operation the after condition would have been much better, there would be a feeling of resentment against the surgeon who performed the useless vandalism, instead of a sort of hero worship that is the general aftermath of a difficult or peculiar operation.

Nature has been kind to us in the matter of paired organs, for we have two eyes, two ears, two kidneys, two lungs, as we have paired hands and feet, but we need the entire equipment if we are to keep well.

It is too much to expect that the young physician will choose the unspectacular role of family physician, or internist, when the prestige is somehow less than the more heroic surgical calling, also not nearly so profitable as the few hours spent daily in the consulting room of the specialist.

Surgery yields large fees, partly determined on the seriousness of the operation and the character of skill required to perform the work, and partially also on the patient's prominence and ability to pay.

If the surgeon operated incognito and for a minimum fee, or a modest fee determined by the government or the governing body of medicine, there would be missing the two prime motives for frequent and difficult operations, and therefore much unnecessary surgery would go undone.

To be either socially prominent or very wealthy greatly increases the liability to frequent and needless surgery, for both social prominence and wealth offer great temptation to the ambitious surgeon, and most surgeons are ambitious, or I read them all wrong.

In the matter of appendicitis alone, during twenty-six years past, no case going through the writer's hands has required operation, nor was any surgeon permitted to consult with such case. Up to date no deaths have occurred from this bloodless treatment; more than four hundred cases of every type of the condition having recovered easily and very quickly, simply through emptying the colon, withholding of everything from the digestive tract, and the application of the simple ice bag. This number includes nineteen cases in which rupture had already occurred before the case came under treatment. Until one case is lost through this simple and safe form of management it is not surprising that he refuses to be frightened by any type of appendicitis.

Yet the surgeon who is told that there is a possibility of spontaneous cure without surgery will bend on his informer a look of the deepest pity, for he thoroughly believes in the essentially surgical character of this condition, as he believes in the immortality of his own soul, or the infallibility of his past experience.

When any condition as intimately bound up with a surgical conception as is appendicitis can be completely dissociated from all surgical consideration to the number of well over four hundred cases, without one death to argue against this unsurgical conception, surely there must be something wrong with the training of any man who wishes to put every physician in jail for spreading the gospel of sane treatment for such a simple condition. The thing has already become associated so intimately with surgery as to make a consent for operation in any case of appendicitis one of the easiest attacks on the pocketbook that is offered to the hungry surgeon in the entire field of operative possibilities.

Scarcely does a day pass without the record of some case that yesterday was in his usual health, today brings news that he was taken suddenly with an acute attack of appendicitis; his medical advisors fear rupture, rush him to the hospital, operate "in the nick of time," and tomorrow's news chronicles his untimely death. The thing is so common as to excite scarcely two inches of space, and seldom front page, unless the victim is socially prominent or a national figure.

No tonsil is ever so hopelessly diseased as to deserve removal, and one of the largest and best equipped pathological laboratories in this country reports that in one thousand tonsils removed in a short time in the hospital with which this laboratory is connected, examination showed that but seven per cent were actively diseased, and but thirty per cent showed even traces of former disease, now healed.

There is unnecessary surgery, for which someone should be punished, yet there is no way to bring either punishment or damage suit against the surgeon who performs these unnecessary operations.

Education that will be effective in controlling this surgical menace must be directed toward the public; for it is too much to expect that the surgeons will easily forego the lucrative and spectacular exercise of any function that has cost them plenty to acquire and that offers as easy "pickings" as does surgery, whether necessary or not.

And so it all comes back to the fact that we do not individually know enough, not nearly enough, about our own bodies and how they become ill, and this ignorance breeds fear, and we fall easy victims to any form of treatment that we are told is necessary to free us from some impending calamity which we usually only imagine.

The cause of so much surgery may be charged first to this

ignorance and fear on our own part, and scarcely less is it chargeable to the willingness of the surgeon to take advantage of both ignorance and fear in his proposed treatment of us.

The way out is easy enough, if we remember that all of our troubles are self-created, and controllable only through self-management.

To operate is to delete the evidences of a diseased condition that had its beginning away back in our mistaken manner of living, chiefly in our manner of refueling our bodies. Instead of removing an evidence of the former mistakes it is much more to the point to detoxicate, get rid of much of the offending material that has furnished the only possible background for the surgical condition, thus obviating the surgery and at the same time placing the body in such condition as to prevent future occasions for surgical happenings.

This form of treatment costs nothing, it is self-applied, and leads to better instead of worse conditions in after life.

It is possible that because of these very facts the line of treatment which looks toward a better condition of the body is hard to impress as a necessary condition on the mind of most, for it does not cost anything, and it does require self-application, which to most of us is a painful consideration. How we do love to do what we want to do, when we want to do it; and how we love to delude ourselves into thinking that, however we have lived, there is always someone who can get us out of payment for the effects of our foolishness!

To live right, so as to cost us nothing in dissipated vitality, is easier than to live wrong, if we understand the thing thoroughly; and there is infinitely more fun in it.

Instruction in the art of living to keep one hundred per cent well at all times should begin in the early life of the school child. The principles can be easily grasped by the beginner in school, and often more easily than by older ones who have already formed rather fixed habits of eating.

The taking of nourishment and the exercise of the sex function are both fundamental to perpetuation of the race, and both functions should be thoroughly understood early enough in life to avoid the awful consequences of an ignorance that has shortened the life of so many, has defeated every early ambition, brought misery, illness, unhappiness, and too often terminated in suicide, all because no one either cared or realized the necessity for special instruction in these two fundamental necessities of living.

Sex life is not to be discussed here, but food will be so thoroughly gone into before the finis is reached that if you are undecided as to how to properly nourish your own body it will not be the fault of this particular writer.

The history of medicine is behind us now, and we will confine all future remarks to the individual responsibility of each reader in the matter of his or her own health, well knowing that science as it has been worked out in laboratories of nutrition will bear out every statement made as to competent nourishment.

All the findings of these laboratories of nutrition have been checked and double-checked on the human in private practice for years.

CHAPTER II.

What Is Health?

WE are too apt to think of health as something that simply happens, something for which we are perhaps truly thankful, but oftener something that we accept as one of the happenings of nature, and for which we take neither credit nor responsibility.

Through good heredity we do inherit health to some degree, but far more do we create health by living within the immutable laws of chemistry.

The best heredity may be rapidly dissipated through unwise management of our body powers and exceeding our body capabilities, or neglecting to replenish fully our body's own losses.

Perfect health is nothing but one hundred per cent function of every organ and tissue of the body. Some have more health than others, but we all have health, else we would not be alive. Health is function, and function is life, and without function there is no life; so, again I say, we all have health.

If health is one hundred per cent function, that is, perfect health, then everything below this is disease; for disease is never anything else than deficiency of health, no matter what symptoms it manifests, nor what its myriad modes of expression.

Both health and disease are relative terms; neither can ever be absolute, for the healthiest individual in the world will always have some evidences of conditions less than health; neither can the sick man be one hundred per cent sick, for that would mean complete absence of function, or death. As we function less than normal in any particular we are to exactly that same percentage sick, or less than well.

The creation of health, as well as its maintenance, is wholly a matter of keeping up body function, and this can be done without the least difficulty, given the right foods used in the right way, and an ordinary amount of the other adjuvants to health in the form of air, sun, exercise, sleep and play, for play has its place in health, just as surely as does the sun, even though not to the same extent.

Nature provides a self-governing mechanism for the maintenance of health, or function, but this presupposes certain natural conditions that will allow freedom from any deterring influences that could in any way interfere with nature's work. In exactly so far as we allow nature free and unhampered play for her direction of body function will she work to the best advantage in creating and maintaining health, or function.

Savage and uncivilized races, without literature to guide them, have none of the diseases of civilization, simply because they do not have the deterrent customs and environment of the more highly civilized, thus allowing nature more freedom in carrying out her processes completely.

Col. Robert McCarrison, of the British Army Medical Service, while on duty at a distant post situated in the Himalaya region of India, said that in the nine years he was stationed there he had not come into contact with any case of appendicitis, gastric or duodenal ulcer, gall stones, colitis, constipation, catarrh, indigestion, pyorrhoea, asthma, gout, rheumatism, or any of the other usual pests of civilization, and all his surgical work, except for accidental injuries, was confined to the post itself, with its civilized English habits of life.

The natives were restricted by religious dogma to the outgrowth of the ground for food, with the exception of milk and cheese, of which these people used but little, their chief diet being vegetables, fruits, nuts and whole grain breads. They had no means of refining these simple natural products of the ground, so could not suffer from the usual line of deficiency diseases brought about by our highly civilized habits of refining everything that will lend itself to this wasteful process.

These simple people of the Himalaya region were poor,

[32]

very poor indeed, and it was difficult for each to provide enough food for the members of his family, and everyone worked, else he could not live.

Dr. McCarrison says that the older men of the tribe looked so much like the younger men that he was often not able to tell the one from the other as they worked in the field, or as they swam in the river at the end of the day.

They reported great ages, such as we would not easily believe, but which Col. McCarrison accepted as genuine, after living among these people for nine years.

The older men were apparently as efficient as those of much lower age, and took part in the wrestling and other strenuous sports of the tribe and held their own with the younger men.

It is not hard to find the reasons for this superb condition of these simple people, for their daily food contained everything required by the body at work, play or rest, all in its natural form, except the bread, which was baked, but in its unrefined state this contained still the natural ingredients of the whole grain.

Their life was that of the agrarian, spent outdoors, at active manual labor, so oxidation was insured, with little liability of accumulation of the usual unoxidized waste from which we suffer so much in our unwise eating habits.

They were spared the enervating pleasures that go with the highly civilized, for they were not only too poor to indulge in anything of the kind, but their segregation saved them from contact with the enervating pleasures of the more refined English, or those East Indian localities brought most thoroughly under English habit.

We are not saying anything against English habit, which is on the whole as good as our boasted American habit, and better in one particular, at least, and this is the particular of daily exercise, walking or riding horse-back, golf, tennis, and all out-door sports, of which the English are very fond.

In one particular they are not so fortunate as we, and this

is in the matter of food; for we are becoming a nation of vegetable and fruit-eaters, while the Englishman is still content with his gooey puddings and his afternoon starchy teas.

His larger consumption of starchy foods and meats is largely offset by his greater outdoor activity, but he still exhibits the worst teeth of any nation; a double set of store teeth being very common in the early thirties among the English men and women, while in America this occurs in the late fifties, as a rule.

Nature struggles with might and main to keep us well at all times, and fails only because we have thrown in her way too many impediments in the form of wrong foods, deficient foods, imbalanced foods, refined foods, too much food, insufficient exercise, sun, sleep, play, and because we too long have forgotten that we are made of the dust of the earth, and from the earth must we be nourished.

The sixteen elements and their salts, of which every type of living creature is composed, are all found in the soils of the earth, and from these we absorb everything we need. These elements are used by plant, nut, grain, fruit, changed into colloids and prepared for restoration of our bodies to the normal every night while we sleep.

We can get these same elements second hand if we eat of the fauna that has subsisted on these same vegetable outgrowths of the ground; but to do so fully we are under compulsion of eating the entire animal, else we will again run into deficiencies, and ultimately develop one of the host of deficiency diseases; in other words, a degeneration of the body.

There is no magic by which we are to maintain health, nor any royal road to this; and when we analyze the thing we are compelled to say that all we can do to keep well is to quit making ourselves sick.

Now this all leads up to a fundamental statement that must be the key note throughout this discussion: The only constructive treatment for disease of any kind is to cease causing disease.

We would all be well and always well if we did not continually interfere with nature's own chosen processes, as we do by wrong habit, chiefly wrong ideas of what the body requires in the way of replacement material; food, in other words.

If no other statement of all contained in this volume sticks in your memory, the writer will feel amply repaid if this one has so deeply impressed itself on the cortex of your brain that not all the sophistries of medicine or accepted theory of disease and its treatment can erase the impression — all we can do about disease is to stop causing it.

As remarked before, all medical treatment is directed against disease per se, and no account is taken of the chemical background from which all disease must emanate, if it materializes at all. Yet nothing constructive can be done for disease except to correct this background from which it grows; every other effort being in the nature of a meaningless gesture.

To be sure, much can be done to change symptoms, to bring ease out of pain, to make the body comfortable, but none of these things are constructive treatment, as they do not change the condition that permitted the body to depart so far from health.

To preserve health is to husband our greatest capital, our potential enjoyment and accomplishment throughout a life that may be as long as we wish, if we continue always to cease interference with natural processes, and allow nature to work with us unhampered, as in the case of the East Indian tribe already referred to.

Dr. McCarrison tells us that these men are of exceptional physical beauty, as of course they should be, with small waist, large chest, erect stature, suppleness in every movement, for they are not loaded up with the mass of acid end-products of the less fortunate man who has to contend daily with our hampering customs of civilization.

[35]

To maintain perfect health it is not necessary to forego one of the real pleasures of life, and especially of the pleasures of the table, for food can be more entrancingly enjoyable, if of right sort taken in right manner, than the most epicurean catering of the most up-to-date hostelry, if we only understand the fundamentals of eating.

Food should be replacement material first, enjoyable second, and combined with due regard to the immutable laws of the chemistry that forms us and that can maintain us continually at a high level of efficiency and enjoyment.

So let us admit that food is an important consideration in our daily living, and resolve to understand our body needs as well as we can, arranging our daily intake of food so as to meet these three requirements—the natural character of the foods, their appeal to our aesthetic sense, and their correct combination; and when we have well learned our lesson we can give Epicurus himself cards and spades and beat him out in the final draw.

Do not ask your doctor to subscribe to any such strange beliefs as that one's health is in one's own hands, and that all that is constructive in the treatment of disease is to cease to cause the thing treated, for he will not take kindly to such theory, as his whole training has been along the lines of treatment for disease, and he will be putting himself in the position of one who is tampering with disease instead of eradicating it.

Health is generally considered one thing, disease another; yet I am sure it is not difficult to see that both are differing degrees of exactly the same thing — function, good or bad function.

Given the right kind of food, eaten in the right way, with due respect to the laws of chemistry, in right amount, and with the adjuvants to health provided by nature, then nothing but health can be the result, naturally; for when you have fulfilled the necessary conditions for health, nature would have to suspend some of her immutable laws if anything less than health were to be the outcome.

This does not mean that at once health results, when the requirements for this are fully met, but that the way is now opened for health, or perfect function, and health will grow just as disease formerly grew from the opposite conditions.

While it may require many years to create such a departure from normal health as will express itself in the form of some recognizable disease, yet nature will require but a small part of the time to rebuild.

It is thus that nature works continually for us, and is an evidence of the fact that so long as we live just so long does nature keep up this fight for right conditions. When the fight stops, so do we stop; for this is the end, and function is finally suspended.

Knock off a finger nail and you will replace this in kind in a few weeks or very few months, as we know. Cut the hair and it grows soon to its original length. Abrade the skin on the surface of the body and it is soon replaced with new skin that is exactly like the old, unless the abrasion has been so deep as to involve the lower layer, from which the superimposed layers are replaced, and then nature does the very best she can with what is left, for she builds into the abraded area scar tissue that does very well, but that is not true skin, having neither pores nor hair roots, but nature's patch for material gone and forgotten.

These evidences of growth, rehabilitation, repair, are sure signs that nature is repairing us as best she can continually, and it is our part to see that she is not hampered in her work.

Just as the external parts are replaced and repaired, even so surely are the internal parts also replaced and repaired daily, yearly, throughout our entire lives.

We die daily, and daily we are reborn, cell by cell, till the entire body has been changed in time into a new body; one that

may be well or less than well, depending wholly on how we
have provided for this rebirth.

Cells of some of the special organs are of very short life,
the red cell of the blood being about two weeks old when it
again breaks up and is replaced with a new cell.

Bone cells are supposed to be of long life, as also the cells
of the brain and nerve tissue. In fact, scientists are quite of
the opinion that the cells of the brain are lifelong, those with
which we were born being still with us when we die. If this is
true it will easily account for the fact that of all the diseases
of the body only those of degeneration of nerve cells and tissues
do not respond to regenerative eating, but tend to continue their
degenerative course to final paralysis.

All the catarrhal and inflammatory conditions to which the
organs and tissues of the body are subject, tend to get well
when relieved of the irritation of acid end-products, through
detoxication and such dietary correction as will end the production of these irritants in excess of what can be eliminated
daily and fully.

Thus, again, all we can do constructively for disease is to
stop causing it, for nature will at once begin to repair the
damage done, if not continually hampered by these acid end-
products.

When we knock off the finger nail we do not expect this
at once to be replaced by a new nail, for we recognize the fact
that nature has to go through her processes of repair before
the new nail can appear; but we do recognize the fact that if
ever we are to have a new nail we must refrain from repeat-
edly hitting it with the hammer. Is it not so?

So long as we do the body no harm it remains well, and all
we can do to keep it well is to continually refrain from doing
it harm. This is the law, and we cannot escape its exactions.

Perfect health is not compatible with anything less than
perfect function, which means that no fatigue, no disease, no
headaches, no blues, no depressing emotions are to be found

[38]

combined with perfect health, and when one of these little annoyances is present we are to that extent separated from ideal health.

It is not strange that the doctor is not interested in health, for health is the direct antithesis of everything on which he has concentrated his best thought, and his interest must always be in disease, the opposite of health.

And so the patient is interested in his health, the doctor in his disease, and the interests of these two must always conflict. The patient believes he is less than well because of some accidental happening to his normal functioning; not realizing that all that can happen to normal function does so through the body's own creation of acid end-products of digestion and metabolism. This is something with which the doctor has nothing to do, for all he is trained to do is to treat your diseases, your evidences of disease. It is your particular responsibility to prevent the creation of every deterrent to perfect function, and only you can do this.

If your nutritional state comes from what you eat and how you eat this, then just so surely as no one can eat your food for you, no one can digest it, absorb it, assimilate it, metabolize it but yourself, and no one can keep you well but your own sweet self. It is your job to keep well, and it is the doctor's job to do the best he can to relieve you when you are sick. Your job leaves off just where the doctor's job begins, but if you have done yours well the doctor will never have anything at all to do for you.

It is to impress this fact that this little book is written, and to point the easy way in which this can be accomplished.

If you eat those foods required by the body for replenishment, in their natural form so far as possible; if you take those of unrefined character that chiefly appeal to your sense of taste and enjoyment; if you combine these with due respect to their chemical requirements; then, even if you do neglect exercise, sun, air, rest, play, you can keep reasonably well. But if you do make use of all the other adjuvants named and at the same time you eat wrong foods or denatured foods, or take your foods in incompatible relation, it will be impossible for you to keep well, and the mortician will get you before nature ever intended him to make your acquaintance.

So do not be surprised if the idea is strongly stressed throughout this discussion that foods are of paramount importance in every consideration of health or disease. It is not with the intention of belittling these other very important adjuvants that this is so stressed; for it has been the writer's experience that when people are fed correctly all the other adjuvants to health come to them without any direction from anyone, just as the healthy animal cavorts and plays when in good health, lies in the sun, loves the outdoors.

Get right inside first by nourishing the body competently and keeping elimination up to date, and the rest will so largely take care of itself that it may safely be allowed to do so.

To be in full health is to be free from fatigue, disease, blues, all hampering emotions; and why should you not then indulge in play? You could not be kept from play if healthy enough.

Let us first of all learn correct nutrition; then let us take advantage of every adjuvant to health that nature offers, as we will if the first requisite has been intelligently met and faithfully carried out, and we will soon forget the fatigue, disease of all kinds, and actually enter into a new world of enjoyment and accomplishment.

For this privilege we need thank no one but Mother Nature herself, for it is she that has provided such for us.

CHAPTER III.

How Do We Depart From Health?

THE infant, born into the world complete, is a potential adult, capable of growing into a perfect adult if all the laws of being and of growth are fully complied with continually. But if these laws are spurned, as is usual, deficiencies are developed that may make of the child a delicate specimen, incompletely developed, perhaps deficient in mentality, subject to all the diseases that lie in wait for those who cannot resist. It is not strange that two hundred thousand of these infants in our country never see the end of their second year, that four hundred thousand die before the end of the tenth year, and that seventy-five per cent of American childhood is afflicted with major or minor ailments that class them with the defectives. The children in both urban and district schools are found to be defective in some or many particulars to the extent of seventy-five per cent.

We are a supposedly enlightened and cultured people, possessed of wealth, refinement, advancement in arts and manufacture to such a point that we announce to the world that we are the most enlightened people on earth; yet we have the highest infant mortality of any civilized nation on the earth, and our maternal mortality is far greater than that of any other.

Any infant, born complete, is capable of developing into a perfect adult, no matter what the heredity; for heredity has done all it can do when the birth occurs; and the after care determines the development, whether this be complete or deficient.

After birth the feeding determines the growth and development. Nothing else does; for, in the midst of the most uncongenial surroundings, infant life will develop into perfection, if fed right. Conversely, the infant reared amidst the most perfect surroundings, with the highest type of medical care,

[41]

will develop defectively if not fed correctly, as we all know. The feeding is the thing that determines the after condition, whether in infant life or after adulthood is reached.

Extreme poverty is no excuse for deficient feeding of either adult or infant; for the right foods cost no more than the wrong sort. It is more a question of understanding foods and selecting those that nourish competently, at the same time respecting the laws of chemistry, that determine the resultant nutrition.

Food should represent all the chemical elements of structure and function; twelve of these representing structure, and four representing function only; catalysts, in other words. Not one of these is unimportant to either growth or function, and growth comprehends also rehabilitation or repair; for we never cease to grow, albeit we do cease to increase in stature.

More infantile deficiencies occur from deficient feeding than from any other cause. By deficient feeding we do not mean total deficiency, but specific deficiency, meaning that some necessary elements are either wholly missing or deficient in amount. So that no matter how much so-called food the infant may consume the result may be deficiency, through paucity of some one or more elements.

Overfeeding and incompatible mixtures, with introduction of starches and sugars before the teeth are all developed, perhaps, are second in importance; for these also unbalance nutrition, causing plethoras as well as deficiencies.

If the food is lacking in one element there is soon created a deficiency in some recognizable form, the chief and most common one being rickets, or rachitis, which occurs in the children of the wealthy and enlightened somewhat more frequently than in the children of the under-priviliged and poor; showing that it is not a case of poverty, but one of not knowing how to feed the child.

Fortunately, nature provides perfect food for all her children, no matter in what section of the globe they may reside;

and for each location there grows a profusion of food suitable for sustenance of the fauna of that particular locality.

Thus the children of the frozen north need plenty of fats for fuels during the cold weather, and there is the whale and seal and other fat fish or animals to furnish this necessary fuel.

The children of the sunny south need the fresh fruits and vegetables and there these are found in profusion.

In the temperate zones we have everything necessary for the heat of summer and the cold of winter, all growing out of the ground in the greatest profusion, ready to use.

Civilization has so changed, refined, processed, preserved, beautified, and adulterated our foods that little remains of the original intent of nature; so we in the midst of profusion of foods are too often suffering from deficiencies; starving in the midst of plenty.

Disease attacks only deficient tissues, which may be broadly stated as an incontrovertible fact. We become diseased because we have not the functional activity to resist the encroachment of such things as extraneous germs, accumulation of debris within ourselves, the rigors of cold, the fatigue of work, or the stress of nerve exhaustion.

It is truthfully said that cancer never attacks a healthy tissue; and the same may as truthfully be said of every disease; for the resistent body will not harbor infections, as it will not degenerate in structure or function. The well body degenerates only as it becomes no longer able to cope with the rising tide of its own debris, the acid end-products of digestion and metabolism.

If this is true, then it must be true that if there is no accumulation of these irritating acid end-products there can be no functional failure to cause decline in health.

A certain amount of these acid end-products is the result of the body's own decomposition and death, as the individual cells die and are replaced by other cells; and as these cells die they give off their debris, which is of acid character.

[43]

However, this is so small and unimportant a part of the accumulation of this class of debris, that if this were all we had to take care of, it would be easy to keep the tissues clear continually, as the normal eliminative channels are capable of eliminating a great excess of the ashes or end-products of body activity.

By far the greatest share of these acids develop from the wrong type of foods, or the wrong combinations of even the right types; so acid accumulation is very largely a matter of what we eat and how we combine this.

Protein foods, such as meats, eggs, fish, and cheese, when oxidized, leave behind the greatest amount of the most irritating debris, and we need so little of this class of foods that it is easy to overdo our needs. That we do overdo them is evident from the great mass of protein debris eliminated daily. The average American habit comprises practically ten times as much protein as is required for tissue replacement, and that is all that protein is for, as it is a very poor fuel on which to support activity, expensive in every sense of the term.

The soft tissues of the body, the muscles, glands, nerve tissue, blood vessels, digestive tract, all are built out of protein; so as the cells die they must be replaced in kind, which means that we do need and positively must have enough protein for this purpose, but that is all.

Now when we eat so much more than we need, what becomes of the unneeded part? If it could be easily eliminated it would do us no harm; but, unless we are extremely active, burning up or oxidizing our waste quite completely, this protein does not reach the form of its final ash, urea, but stops as a sub-oxidation ash, a partially converted or imperfectly consumed ash, which is represented by a large array of very acid and very irritating salts, chief of which is uric acid; after which follow a long line of acid urates, xanthin, hypoxanthin, creatin, creatinin, and a host of others, all acid, all irritating, all clinkers, all a monkey wrench in our machinery. It is excess of protein consumption that possibly stands first as a cause of early departure from health.

If we eat less meat, eggs, fish, and cheese, we shall suffer much less from acid creation; and if we exercise far more than most do we shall at least oxidize this excess better and eliminate it better; for the final ash, urea, is easily eliminated in large quantity, while the sub-oxidized debris is difficult of elimination.

Another cause for this departure from health is no doubt the very free use of the refined and thoroughly denatured things, such as white flour preparations, white sugar, refined starches or sugars of any kind.

These are acid forming in high degree, for their oxidation releases carbonic acid in the system, although their debris is not of such irritating or toxic character as that from the protein group. Their chief danger lies in the fact that they do not leave behind in the system enough of the natural alkalin elements, thus predisposing to acid states. So, if we would escape this form of acid autotoxicosis, we will refrain from use of the refined starches and sugars, and adhere to the whole, unrefined sort.

The third usual source of acid formation, through which we saturate ourselves and so depart from perfect function or perfect health, is through disregard for the laws of chemistry as these apply to the digestion of our foods. If all the causes other than this are neglected, adherence to the laws of chemistry in selecting and combining the foods will bring such regeneration in a few weeks as to thoroughly convince the most skeptical that as we eat even so are we.

When we eat starches or sugars, the so-called carbohydrate foods, we have set the stage for a wholly alkalin type of digestion, as this class will not digest in the presence of any acid whatever. Our laboratory work will have taught us this, for we have long since made the test, if we have ever enjoyed the privileges of even the high school lab.

[45]

Saliva is needed for the first step in starchy digestion, and its action is due to a little ferment called ptyalin, which will act in nothing less than a positive alkalinity. Even a neutral medium will negative its action. Without the stimulation of this alkalin medium there is no action of the ptyalin on carbohydrate foods.

So when you eat the starchy bread or baked potato together with an acid fruit, you have taken away the necessary alkalin conditions on which the ptyalin depends, and it will not act, so the starch goes into the stomach unsplit. As there is no ferment in the stomach that can act on starches, these lie undigested, and ultimately pass into the small intestine, where again there is no means for their splitting, they are little or not at all digested, and are sure to ferment in the presence of heat and moisture.

Now the protein foods, such as meats, eggs, fish, or cheese, depend on the action of the pepsin of the gastric juice for their first step in digestion. As pepsin will act in nothing less than a positive acidity, we are up against it if we have eaten largely of starchy foods at the same meal, for the starches require alkalin conditions and the proteins require acid conditions. Your stomach cannot be both things at the same time, for no fluid can be at the same time both acid and alkalin, no more than a room can at the same time be both light and dark. So the gastric juice begins to contain acid for the digestion of the protein, as it must, and away go the alkalin conditions necessary for the digestion of the starchy food, and fermentation sets in, with its formation and release of the fermentation acids.

Here, then, are three ways by which we depart from health, and they are all sources directly related to the food and our manner of combining it. They are self-created, therefore self-controllable only and all the time.

It is through acid formation chiefly that we depart from health, and this is so because of our functional activity, with

[46]

deficient alkalin reserve in the body, or the presence of a considerable amount of free alkali with which the acids are combined. If we had no alkalin reserve to bind these acids as they form we would not live long enough to make a will, for acid is intolerable in the body, and whenever it forms there must be present in the tissues or the fluids of the body sufficient free alkali to at once bind the acids or we would not live. So we are in the habit of saying that functional activity is well proportioned to the size of our alkalin reserve.

When we eat natural foods in their natural form we are not troubled with acid formation, as nature balances these foods very nicely for our digestive ability. But when we introduce the concentrated starches and concentrated proteins we are predisposing ourselves to excessive acid formation, as these are all acid-forming foods. When we eat together these dissimilar foods we make it impossible to even digest them completely, as they are incompatible in simultaneous digestion.

Anything that depletes our alkalin reserve, therefore, is depleting our functional activity, which is our health spelled large.

So the less acid we form the less alkalin reserve will be tied up, and the more perfect will be our function. Also, the less alkalin ash we introduce with our foods the less will be present for the purpose of neutralizing or binding our acid formation. Either horn of the dilemna is sufficient to reduce our functional activity; our health, in other words.

All the vegetables, all the fruits, some of the nuts, all the raw vegetable salads, leave behind an alkalin ash, or base, while all the starches and all the sugars, as well as all the concentrated proteins, the meats, eggs, fish and cheese, leave behind an acid ash. Therefore, the more we eat of the vegetables, salads and fruits, and the less we eat of the proteins or starches, the concentrated foods, the easier it is to maintain a competent

[47]

alkalin reserve, and never forget that this means also a competent functional activity.

The proper proportion of acid-forming foods to base-forming foods, is two parts of the former to eight of the latter, that is, one fifth only of our daily foods should represent the concentrated things, the breads, starches, sugars, meats, eggs, fish or cheese, yet the average habit is almost the reverse of this, the concentrated things predominating on most tables, whether at home or in public eating places.

Four-fifths of the daily foods should consist of the base-forming things, the vegetables, raw salads, fresh fruits. With this class may be combined either milk or buttermilk, as the milk is not acid-forming, nor is it base-forming, but it does not digest well with the concentrated things, the starches, sugars and proteins, so should not be used with any other foods except the base-forming vegetables, salads, fruits.

Away goes the old familiar bread and milk of our forefathers. While this is not a serious mistake to combine milk with bread, yet it is far from ideal, and is best left out of the diet, unless one is already quite robust and able to neutralize much acid formation, by great activity, as in children at their usually quite strenuous play.

The practice of most baby specialists of introducing starchy foods before the teeth are all in place is one of the most fertile causes of the frequent fermentations from which children suffer, the bilious attacks, the lack of appetite, the sour vomiting, the eruptions, the irritability, the bed-wetting habit, and the general early formation of acid states, so that the average child by two years of age has already a well developed acidosis.

Nature does not provide enough ptyalin for the splitting of starches and sugars before the teeth are well developed, or till they are all in place, as a rule, so it is plain that nature intended the child to subsist on the mother's milk for this interval, and provides the ptyalin only when concentrated starches can be thoroughly chewed, which we know to be the very first consideration in their digestion. Without thorough chewing and insalivation the concentrated starches are much better left out of the diet of everyone, for they make too much trouble otherwise.

Before the teeth are in place the concentrated starches and cane sugars are never thoroughly split, and their imperfect digestion is the chief cause of the frequent illnesses of children. These do more to buy gasoline for the baby specialists than almost all the other causes of illness among children. Why impose on the undeveloped digestion of the infant a task that requires adult development of digestion to properly handle?

Little children, before the end of the second year, need nothing but milk. If the mother cannot nurse her child the best substitute is goat milk, and the next best, bovine milk, modified to as near the human standard as possible by dilution to reduce the protein or casein, adding cream to make up for the dilution of the fats, also milk sugar to make up for the dilution of this. The milk should be always raw, for a pasteurized milk has lost its water-soluble vitamines, and is in no sense a complete food. If nothing but pasteurized milk can be obtained, then orange juice should be added to the daily diet, to supply these water-soluble vitamines, for without these there will be neither growth nor health. Orange juice added to the diet of even the breast-fed infant is a wise precaution, for few mothers have all the elements necessary in their milk, from their own deficient habits of feeding previously.

Goat milk is naturally very high in fats, so if diluted half and half with sterile water it needs no addition of cream, and perhaps none of the milk sugar. It is also safest, especially as the goat is not subject to the usual bovine diseases, nor has it been exploited by the veterinarian as has the cow, and for this reason is apt to give more nearly a natural milk. Tuberculin testing of cattle introduces a hazard, for only since this practice became quite universal have we heard of undulant fever, contagious abortion, and other diseases of the milk cow.

[49]

When the infant is six months of age it is safe to introduce puréed vegetables, as spinach, turnip, beet, carrot, celery, even cabbage. The purée may be given in small amount and increased as well borne, to a tablespoonful once or even twice a day, at the same time increasing the milk as the baby grows, and adding fruits of other sorts, as tomato, ripe and raw, which is almost as good as the orange juice.

Scraped apple may be given early, perhaps as early as the purée of vegetables; but reliance should be placed on the juice of the orange for the water-soluble vitamines so necessary for growth and development.

As much as an ounce or more of orange juice may be used an hour before each nursing or feeding, if the baby likes this, and almost all babies seem to have a natural fondness for orange juice.

The sun bath should not be neglected, and can be given daily; even in cold weather the baby may be wrapped warmly and set out on the verandah for air and sun during sleep.

This is all to start the first year right; and if proper attention is given to the feeding during this first year all goes well as a rule, unless the mother listens to some of her neighbors or to her doctor, and introduces starchy foods before the end of the second year.

As growth occurs, any food that is good for the adult is good for the baby of more than two years, for the needs are the same.

There will be no departure from health if such feeding habits persist till growth is well on the way, and when the teeth are developed for chewing a variety of foods.

Now, to recapitulate, let us go back over the causes that produce the decline in alkalin reserve, which are the causes of ill health, or the departure from health, rather.

First, the use of entirely too much protein food, in the form of meats, eggs, fish, or cheese; second, the use of the refined, denatured, starchy, or sweet foods, the sugars and starches that make up so much of the average diet; third, the use of incompatible mixtures of food, as those of starchy or sweet sort combined with either the acid fruits or the proteins, such as meat or eggs.

These three food causes combine to produce enough acid end-products to seriously tie up our alkalin reserve, thus lowering function, and interfering with health. which is merely normal function.

Now we depart from health in just the proportion to which we have allowed our alkalies to be dissipated by introduction of acid-forming food in too great amount. This is an easily controllable factor, and when controlled there ceases to be decline in our alkalin reserve and we begin to see a departure of all the former evidences of disease.

If the student of foods will attack this last cause first, it will easily prove the correctness of the whole theory; for this one care alone will produce such a change in feelings as will easily convince the most skeptical of the great necessity for conservation of a proper alkalin reserve.

When these incompatibilities are cut out of the eating habit there is so much alkali conserved that the effect of this is felt easily within the first two weeks. I have frequently challenged the unbelieving to make this test, and have yet to find one who will make it honestly and painstakingly who will not admit that it made a great change in the feelings in this short time.

The separation of the incompatible foods also automatically cuts down the consumption of both proteins and starches, for each type is thus limited to less meals per day than formerly, so helping in this particular as well as in limiting the acid formation through making the digestive tasks all compatible.

It is rare indeed to find anyone who will make this change for two weeks who will not continue to do this as a habit afterward, and with surprising results in regeneration, and disap-

[51]

pearance of many former annoying symptoms and conditions that were not pleasant.

To separate the incompatible foods is to continue to eat just the same things as formerly, but in different groupings, that is all. This is no difficult program, and entails no real self-denial, so should be undertaken easily by anyone, even the confirmed devotee of the table.

When the sun shines brighter, the birds sing more sweetly, the day passes without the usual irritations, the former fatigue is less in evidence, then you will know that your alkalin reserve is rising, and it will not be difficult for you to persuade yourself that somehow you are on the right track at last. A continuance of this habit of separating your incompatible foods will seem not only no hardship, but rather an addition to the usual pleasures of life, for all will be heightened by an even slight increase in the alkalin reserve.

There will be slight loss of weight, perhaps, at first, as the body rearranges its stores and cleans house of the former acid excess, but this is merely an adjustment period through which the body must pass before coming into a better condition. The ultimate result will be gain in weight if you are now too low, just as it will be loss of weight if you are of the obese type, the tendency of the body being always toward the normal when the excessive acid formation is stopped and function can again begin to resume its normal.

This is a consummation devoutly to be wished by both the thin and the obese; for both conditions are evidence of abnormal states of body chemistry. And remember that all these aberrations of body chemistry are due to retention of the acid end-products of digestion and metabolism, and you will understand why this program will make you better.

CHAPTER IV.

The Effect of Food on the Mind

A T first glance no connection between food and thinking is apparent; yet I assure you that just so surely as food affects the body it also affects our thinking, for the very same reasons as pertain to the body. Our thought processes are influenced directly by what we have eaten; perhaps not from what we have last eaten, but surely from what we eat habitually.

The brain is given credit with the processes of thought, though some profess to doubt this, and maintain that thought originates outside us, in the ethereal universe. But wherever it originates, the processes are as certainly run by the body, some part of the body, as that our digestion, circulation, breathing, are functions of the body; and as the brain occupies the most strategic position in the body for direction of impulses everywhere, it is the logical seat for emotions, motivating impulses, and conscious thinking.

The brain is the great reflex center, from which radiate all nerves that control motion and sensation; and as the brain must depend on the body for blood and oxygen, surely it must be affected by what we eat; for what we eat determines the sort of blood we have.

A brain nourished by blood laden with all sorts of acid debris is surely not in condition or position to function at its highest best. And thus it works out; for toxic states may so befuddle the brain that clear thinking is impossible, and even deep comatose states will result from unusually deep types of intoxication, as we often observe.

If we are unable to breathe for three or four minutes we become unconscious, comatose, because the blood, unable to make the eighteen-times-a-minute exchange between carbon dioxide and oxygen, is in a deeply toxic state, poisoned by carbon dioxide retention.

This phenomenon we see in drowning or suffocation, and recognize the character of the intoxication as carbon dioxide poisoning.

If carbon retention will in three or four minutes produce this serious poisoning, then why will not retention of other deleterious toxins do the same thing, though not so quickly?

When the body begins to detoxicate, to throw off the saturation with acid end-products of digestion and metabolism, one of the first observable effects is a clearing up of dull mental states, and an ability to think far more clearly than formerly. The less toxic the body the clearer the brain, as we are able to observe in numberless cases; and, conversely, the deeper the type and degree of intoxication, the duller the mentality.

As said before, one of the earliest evidences of a lessening of the toxic state is a mental improvement, long before there is any physical improvement in sight, showing that the brain responds to the detoxication before the body does.

This is to be expected, for structurally there is nothing wrong with the brain, but its function is interfered with by the toxic character of the blood which supplies it with material for the thinking processes, for it has been demonstrated that thinking does take energy, does use up fuels, though not to the same extent as the body.

So, when the blood begins to carry less waste to the brain there should be improvement in thought processes at once. And this is just what happens, while the body has to regenerate from the former depressing effects of the toxic state that has caused much structural change, perhaps. The body has to restore itself to the normal after the toxic state declines, but the brain is normal at once.

There is an improvement in the general feeling that precedes physical improvement, for the reason given; and everyone who has gone through the detoxication period preceding a proper dietary correction, can testify to this fact.

The evidences of failure of the brain are slow thinking,

poor reasoning power, loss of memory, lack of power to concentrate; and of these, the last named is surely one of the most
marked.

The writer well remembers that before his break-down
twenty-six years ago last winter, he had for a long time been
unable to concentrate fixedly for more than a very few
moments; and to read through and appreciate any scientific
article was almost a lost art with him for three or four years
past. Yet in two weeks from the beginning of his dietary
change he was able to think for long periods fixedly on one subject, and was able to read through and well evaluate scientific
articles that for a long time past might just as well have been
written in Sanskrit.

With the returning mental alertness and ability to concentrate there developed a certainty of coming improvement in
every way, and soon optimism took the place of pessimism.
A memory that before was so deficient that even an ordinary
conversation was a painful proceeding, developed a prompt-
ness that was astonishing; facts seemingly long forgotten were
available for instant use; and now, after this rather long period,
public speaking is never fraught with any misgivings, for
memory is instantaneous, and seldom is it necessary to pause
for word or fact during an address of thirty minutes to an
hour or more.

He has long since passed the age when one is supposed to
have said goodbye to his prime, yet memory is better each year;
active sports, such as tennis and golf, are thoroughly enjoyed
any day; and in tennis, which is a quite active game for those
in fine physical condition, his game is fully as good as it was
forty years ago, perhaps better. Age has seemed to stand still,
or even recede, for the past twenty-five years.

He knows of others who, after even longer periods, and
at a more advanced age, are improving physically and mentally still; one of the most striking cases being that of
Dr. Robert G. Jackson, of Toronto, Ontario, who at forty-nine

years of age was given up to early death, with Bright's disease, high blood pressure, hardening arteries, double glaucoma, haemorrhage into the base of one eye that had completely obliterated the sight, and neuritis and arthritis that had made him a cripple for five years before he began a regenerative way of eating that has led him back to better conditions with each year. Now he is fit continually at seventy-five years, athletic, able to run ten miles every day, erect as a soldier, (instead of bent double as formerly), and has two perfectly good eyes.

Dr. Jackson tells the writer that he is every year able to do things that he could not do the year before, or to do the same things better than the year before; and his condition today is like that of a young man in his twenties; an athletic young man at that.

So does nature work for us instead of against us, when we cease to interfere with her processes.

The writer has listened to Dr. Jackson talk for an hour and a half without the slightest hesitation for a word, and exhibit all the mental and physical alertness of a young man; for he has written the word fatigue out of his lexicon, and never suffers from that inhibiting sensation either day or night.

When you consider his low beginning, a physician who was a teacher of medicine in a Philadelphia medical college who knew plenty about disease, but could not save himself from degeneration, with one of the worst family histories imaginable, the oldest member of his family dying at forty-three years of age, and all the others at lesser ages, and all of the same conditions from which he himself suffered, it makes one of the most impressive instances of physical regeneration on record; perhaps it would be safe to say the MOST impressive, for I have never heard of one more striking than Dr. Jackson's own history.

We were talking about the effect of food on thinking, and Dr. Jackson's case came at once to mind, for he had told the writer that his case, like my own, showed first as a lightening of the mental processes as improvement set in. Observation of numberless cases of regeneration has shown quite uniformly this same mental regeneration preceding by usually several days any feeling of physical regeneration; showing that what was said previously is demonstrable; that the brain does not have to recover, as it has undergone no physical changes; and as soon as the depressing toxic state begins to pass, already the brain is again on a higher functional plane.

In public speaking one has to have at his tongue's end so many facts, that if the memory and ability to concentrate are not both working at high speed one might better stay off the platform; for floundering is painful to any audience, and only when the brain is competently nourished can it be as alert as it is supposed to be.

Many are familiar with the sensation of mental fatigue and its paralyzing effects; yet fatigue of either brain or physique comes always and only from a toxic state of the circulation, nothing else.

When muscle breaks down fuels to furnish energy, these fuels, during oxidation, leave behind an acid ash; and if the blood is already well saturated with this sort of debris it is not nascent, not able readily to take up this debris and remove it from the field of activity, and its accumulation there is the sole cause of muscular fatigue. It is even so with the brain; for if its activities must be supported by oxidative processes, then there must be left behind this acid ash, even as in muscular activity, and the circulation must be well freed habitually of this sort of material if it is able to take up quickly and transport to the lungs this acid debris for elimination, thus keeping the field of activity clear, and so preventing the accumulation that spells fatigue.

So it is not difficult to see the connection between foods and mental activity; for even as the body is fatigueless if not intoxicated, just so is the brain, and clear thinking depends

[57]

far more on the right foods eaten in the right way than people dream of in the average philosophy.

It has been said on good authority that mentally we are far more inefficient than physically. Physically we are estimated to be less than half efficient, less than half as efficient as we should be or as we easily can be, and mentally the percentage of efficiency on the average is supposed to be far lower than this.

The cause for this inefficiency is clear, if we keep in mind the few facts recited above; for our thinking depends on the character of feeding habits to an even greater extent than does our physical efficiency. Children of less than average intelligence have been fed correctly and returned to school to lead their classes, because of this improvement in the character of the feeding habit.

Men in business have promoted themselves, have increased their incomes, have accomplished far more than ever before from this same improvement in brain circulation, through right eating; and the number of those who have testified to this is legion.

So, from the standpoint of income alone, it pays big dividends to learn to eat correctly, instead of continuing to make the little foolish mistakes that interfere with brain function just as surely as with physical function of all kinds.

The food for the physical laborer and the brainworker need not differ in character, except as the physical laborer or the one who takes vast amounts of physical exercise needs more of the fuels, in the form of bread, potatoes, cereals, sugars or sweets, for it is these foods that furnish the fuel of which he consumes much in his exercise, while the brain worker consumes far less in the operation of his mental processes. The sedentary man who neither works nor thinks needs but little fuel; and it is a question whether he should have even this small amount, as anything necessary to keep such a one up is wasted, largely.

In manufacturing or mechanics the successful man is he who can make the most out of the least material; and manufacturing economy is one of the great aims of the manufacturer.

We are each a factory, and our output is either mental, thoughts, or physical, deeds, and our necessity for economy is far greater than in the case of the manufacturer.

When we are not suffering from a saturation with end-products we are efficient, both mentally and physically; and when we are loaded with these irritants we are inefficient, subject to fatigue, confusion of mind, indecision, inability to concentrate, or other evidence of mental fatigue.

It is often surprising, after twenty-six years of observation of numberless cases of every type, to see the come-back that almost always starts as a mental uplift, followed by a physical regeneration; for it would seem naturally that the body would show first the evidences of an improving nutrition; while the opposite is the case, the brain showing these evidences first.

A student at college should know the effect of foods on his scholastic standing, as well as on his athletic performance. If right eating will increase and perfect his athletic performance, as it undoubtedly will, it will reflect even more on his scholastic marks.

The usual methods of feeding in college boarding houses are notoriously poor for either athletic or scholastic work; as the average boarding house keeper has fed her boarders wrong during her entire life of service in this line of work that is usually taken incidentally, but which, in point of fact should occupy an important place in every college.

The number of physical and mental break-downs during or soon after a college course, which are many indeed, might be accounted for largely by the classes of foods consumed while studying night and day. No doubt it would be possible to demonstrate this fact by so arranging the feeding habits of an entire college as to show plainly the effects of food on both the physique and the mind of the student at hard work.

Already some few schools are making the attempt to study the effect of food on their student body; but to be scientific these should all be controlled experiments, dividing the boys into two groups, the one fed as per usual and the other fed properly; then the next year the groups switched for comparison, thus making of the experiment one controlled by comparison of these two groups.

If the average university knew the effects of right eating habits on the student body there would occur promptly a great change; nutrition occupying a prominent place, not alone in medical colleges, but in every university department.

It is so easy to demonstrate the effect of foods on endurance, which is an accurate guide to nutrition, that it would be well for every school that has the welfare of the students at heart to start at once a demonstration class to prove the effect of right eating habit on endurance; a thing that can be done easily in any school with the full co-operation of the mass of students.

The word "diet" should never be used; for right eating is in no sense diet; rather it is scientific eating, or eating for a purpose.

In the treatment of many cases, during twenty-two years that have been devoted to sanatorium work on all sorts of cases, the mental uplift reached in two or three weeks to the production of poetry of good standard, from minds that had never before thought in verse. The speech took on a higher plane, as the thoughts were of higher character, and mental development was most striking, as the whole man regenerated.

As the mind is supported by purely physical processes it is not hard to see the connection between foods and thinking; for the physical processes depend so wholly on the character of the body chemistry, and this on the character of foods taken and the manner of combining these, that we cannot seem to dissociate the mind from foods.

[60]

During prolonged fasts, when the body nears an atoxic state, the mind is on such a high level that the subconscious mind becomes very active, and one can almost see through the occult. Some of the greatest mental feats have been performed during prolonged fasts, and a high degree of mental efficiency has been noted for rather long periods following the fast.

Prolonged fasting clears the system of much debris, so of course the brain is nourished with a much purer blood stream, and rises to such heights of efficiency as would not seem possible to one fed ordinarily.

It is said that we never forget any facts that we have ever encountered; that these, when we say they are forgotten, are merely mislaid; that somewhere in the inner consciousness of the subconscious mind these facts are still recorded, and that on favorable occasion, when something happens to suggest them, they will rise again into consciousness, and we say we had forgotten this fact. When the blood stream is well cleared of debris all these forgotten or mislaid facts are again uncovered and ready for instant use; showing that all that was needed to make them again available was a more hygienic state of the body. I am sure we all have noted these experiences, and surely this must be the logical way to account for these facts.

It is surely true that we know little of our mental possibilities till we have furnished the brain with a proper blood supply; and we may not have even touched the possibilities in all our former lives.

It is hard to conceive of the wasted mentality of the toxic, for with a less toxic state so much more could be accomplished that it is a pity indeed that more is not known and practiced of the now well established facts of nutrition. This is a waste incomputable, and as inexcusable as it is preventable.

We have achieved much in mechanics, invention, science; but how much more might we have achieved if we had known the simple facts of a proper nutrition as a background for thinking more efficiently!

The ancient philosophers of Greece placed proper dietary first in training their students, and practiced such rigid economy in the use of foods as shows clearly the importance of this subject in their philosophy.

Epicurus, Socrates, Plato, and many others, placed great stress on food and its manner of use as a background for philosophic study; and themselves practiced what they preached.

The philosophy of these sages stands today on a very high plane after the ages that have passed; and it has been said that some of the utterances of these men contain wisdom that seemed so far in advance of their times as to appear inspired.

Out of a foul body come foul thoughts, and out of a clean body come clean thoughts; so much of the responsibility of our thinking rests on our manner of feeding, however remote the connection may seem to those who have not seen the thing demonstrated in many thousands of cases of various types.

As the body is cleared of acid debris, thinking is at once on a much higher plane; aspiration for the higher things of life is in the foreground; and the baser thinking, the grosser pleasures, seem to be idle and useless—beneath our desire at the time.

"As a man thinketh in his heart so is he," is more than a trite saying, for it is capable of active and most convincing proof. As the body clears of this waste material with which it formerly had been loaded, the mind soars to heights not formerly glimpsed by toxic minds; and new worlds seem to open to the fortunate one.

Most of the worthwhile things of life, those things that have elevated others, that have stood as great accomplishments for ages, have been achieved by those who placed accomplishment before idle pleasure; and among all these benefactors try to find a glutton!

Gluttony and clear thinking, or thinking that has stood for

[62]

ages and is still accepted today as the truth, do not belong together; and the wholly sensuous devotee of the table is bound by his habits to life on a much lower plane than that to which he might easily aspire, if he took food for a purpose, rather than for the sensuous pleasure of eating.

When you hear a man say that he owes his body the best of food you can applaud his wisdom; but make sure that he does not mean lots of the foods he has learned to like, whether these are good for his body or not. Watch him eat, and see if he does not mean that he intends to indulge his pleasures of taste above the other pleasures of life.

The writer has known men who labored with their hands for a small wage, yet who felt that as they were the wage-earners therefore they themselves should have lots of the foods they liked best. And he has seen these same men deny to their families all but the bare necessities of life, while they themselves ate freely of all the good things, as they judged these, and who early in life ate themselves into a condition of such inefficiency that no job was safe for them.

This is a mistaken idea of what we owe to the body; for while we do owe it the best of care, as the temple of God, yet this care is so woefully misunderstood, as a rule, that more harm is done to the body than can be computed, through this same idea of keeping it well fed.

Eating is and should be a science, and one of the greatest importance to all, for it is such a fundamental thing; so much depends on it for our efficiency, health, happiness, accomplishment, that it should have a high place in the early training of everyone.

Yet the opposite of this is true, there being little or no importance attached to it as a study; and the result is that lives are wasted that could have been of infinite service to state and family and self, and life is little enjoyed because of the low plane occupied by those who are weak and inefficient, either mentally or physically.

[63]

Now, if it is becoming clear that the subject of food, as this relates to thinking, is of real importance, then one object of the writer has been fully attained. And if you are not only interested in the thing, but sufficiently impressed to make the experiment before suggested, of complete separation of all incompatibles of the daily foods, then the thing is near proof for you. To make sure that you are on the right track begin at once to separate from each other all those foods of opposite digestive requirements and see what happens.

When you eat your starches or sugars, the so-called carbohydrate foods, do not at the same time take any acid fruits or other acid foods, and no meats, eggs, fish or cheese. Take the carbohydrates at one meal and the proteins and acid fruits at another, and note the change in your thinking and feeling that will follow this one simple test.

If the change is as great as you have been led here to believe, then go the whole distance; make your food intake eighty per cent alkalin or base-forming, by eating vegetables and fruits to the extent of this large percentage every day, and take not more than twenty per cent of the concentrated or acid-forming foods, as the breads, cereals, sugars, meats, eggs, fish or cheese, any or all óf these for the entire day held down to twenty per cent of the entire day's intake, and you will see a still further elevation of mind and feelings, till in time you could not be persuaded to go back to the former heterogeneous mixture of incompatibles and inimicals that we have formerly called a good meal.

This test is open to anyone, it costs nothing, it can do no harm, for it does not change the character or amount of the foods, but simply changes the combination; hence there is no danger in trying it.

CHAPTER V.

The Great American Disease

AMERICA has a disease that may safely be called great, not only because it is nearly universal, but more because its results are so vast. It is not a contagious disease, not transmissible by contact, nor is it one that can be segregated, all alike being exposed to its effects.

It is costing America more every year than the late world war. It is breeding discontent, fear, inertia, blues, headaches, illnesses of all sorts, cutting down the efficiency of the nation needlessly, interfering with individual, state and national programs of every sort; yet it goes unrecognized, unrelieved, almost unnoticed.

But it is curable, wholly so, and this entirely without expense, without legislation specially designed, without national attention, but by a gradual education of the individuals of the nation, and in no other way can the subject be attacked.

If this disease were contagious, if it were subject to quarantine, if it could be met by operation or medication, there would be a great stirring of effort to get rid of this old man of the sea.

We are referring to individual and national fatigue, and to nothing else, for it is well-nigh universal in our fair land. It is costing us infinitely too much, and is making us a near second class nation; yet fatigue is a curable condition, through a simple process of education and the application of a very few rules that do not entail any suffering.

Have you ever reflected on the subject? Have you ever asked yourself why so many people are tired? Have you ever asked yourself why you have been tired when you have done nothing to warrant or account for fatigue? Yet you do get tired; you do get up in the morning with this old man of the sea draped about your shoulders, and you should be rested fully when first arising after a night of presumably refreshing sleep.

It is during sleep that we regenerate, recharge our run down batteries, rebuild the broken defenses. We should be at our best early in the morning, and why is this not so?

Too often we arise, we drag through the first two or three hours of the day, and often do not seem to come to life till the evening offers us amusement of some sort.

We look longingly at the bed and curse fate that we have to go to work, comparing ourselves with the galley slave who is chained to his seat and compelled to work unceasingly.

We wish we might return to the softness of the bed for another forty winks, and we feel driven, compelled, by the necessities of earning a living for ourselves or family.

There is never but one cause for fatigue of this sort and this cause is the inability of the body to eliminate fully every day all the waste products created every day.

There are two kinds of fatigue, the one physiological, the other pathological; the one a natural result of exertion, physical or mental, nature's warning that we have expended enough energy for the time being and must rest till the body has eliminated most of the debris created by our activities; the other, pathological fatigue, a disease, just as definite a disease as smallpox or tuberculosis, one that has not earned its existence through effort, for it is with us almost all the time. This type of fatigue, pathological fatigue, is created in every case by the accumulation of acid end-products of digestion and metabolism, and from nothing else.

You will recall that we stated earlier that this was what disease is; a departure from the normal that is brought about through the creation by and retention in the body of these ashes from foods and from the oxidation of fuels used through activity, yet not excreted as fast as formed; the resulting saturation being the cause of all departures from health, and fatigue is a departure from health, therefore a disease.

[66]

Few are willing to believe that there is such a thing as complete freedom from fatigue, meaning this pathological fatigue which we are discussing. Without the slightest doubt the condition of complete freedom from fatigue can be attained without the least difficulty; not at once, for even if we desist from the creation of excessive amounts of acid end-products, we still must give the body time to fully eliminate the waste now carried. We do not recover at once from disease, but must create the conditions that will permit of recovery and then wait patiently till the body has had time to become normal.

Thus, when we cease the creation of the usual vast amount of acid end-products we usually feel almost at once a great lightening of the mind, and a general feeling of well-being that encourages us to go on; and then we come to a time when we seem to lose this uplifted feeling.

This is because when we cease to eat wrong there is at once a lowering of toxins in the blood stream, which is sure to reflect as a better feeling, a mental uplift, for two to four weeks. But we must remember that the entire body is saturated with this same debris, and as the blood unloads its debris, the body soon comes to give up its own stores to the blood and again a feeling of depression sets in. This may continue for weeks, or occasionally months, with occasional glimpses of the good feeling, till the body has quite unloaded itself, when we soon begin to sense the uplifted feeling most of the time.

When we reach the stage where there is no longer the depression, the discouragement, blues, biliousness, we will know that we are fairly well unloaded; and then we will discover that our former fatigue is entirely gone, we can go on and on all day, keeping busy with whatever is at hand to do, and always without this feeling of fatigue. When intoxication is gone then fatigue is gone; for pathological fatigue is nothing but intoxication; self-intoxication.

In the winter of 1924 the writer was a member of a gymnasium class in the Buffalo Y.M.C.A., and undertook a test of endurance through correcting the diet of eighteen men, ranging in age from 28 to 55 years.

These men were of average dietary habit, average age, average activity, being all professional men except two, who were desk workers.

Their dietary habit was not disturbed except so far as necessary to separate their incompatibles at meals, which allowed them milk and fruit for breakfast, or just fruit, if they did not like milk. Lunch was a starchy type of meal, consisting of bread, vegetables, salads and sweet fruits or ice cream. Dinner was a protein type of meal, consisting of meats, eggs, fish or cheese, with cooked vegetables, raw vegetable salads, fresh acid fruits, and for dessert jello or fruit jello, or sliced acid fruits. No acids were taken at the starch meal, and no starches or sugars with the protein meal, thus separating the incompatible carbohydrates and proteins into two separate meals.

This was all, for no exercise was prescribed, no stimulants or medicines were given, and the men were eating just the same foods as were habitual to them, but in compatible mixture.

They were forbidden to practice the test used, for of course practice would increase endurance. We selected the squat as a fatigue check, as this cannot be faked; the body weighing just so much is lifted from the squat to the upright position as many times as can be accomplished, as a standard, and each week the test is applied to see how many more squats can be performed.

The men were promised fifty per cent increase in endurance at the end of the four week test, during which they were to continue to eat as prescribed and refrain from practicing the squat.

The first week check showed an increase of fifty per cent, and the end of the fourth week showed an increase of one hundred and sixty-five per cent.

This surely would tend to show that the former lack of endurance of these men was due to the accumulation of acid end-products resulting from their incompatible mixtures of dis-similar foods, or those foods that require dissimilar treatment in the stomach; for no change was made in their manner of eating except to separate these known incompatibles.

The causes of fatigue are the causes of disease, nothing more or less. You will remember that we discussed previously the causes of all departures from health, and discovered that they all come from foods, and our mistaken way of treating the daily foods, in the use of far too much protein, the use of the refined and processed starches and sugars, and the incompatible mixture of foods.

You will note that of these three causes we touched only the third, the incompatible mixtures, as this is the one the effect of which is felt at once, while the use of the refined foods can be continued for long periods before the body begins to suffer from deficiencies.

Also, the separation into different groups automatically cuts down the amount of both carbohydrates and proteins, by limiting each to one meal per day. While we stressed only the separation of the incompatibles, yet we also limited the protein, as also the starch, but the effect on endurance was due almost wholly to the separation of the incompatible foods, in this way limiting fermentation with its acid production.

Now here was a direct demonstration of the effect of this separation on endurance; for surely there is no other way to account for this very unusual increase except this one of the arrest of fermentation.

These men are occasionally met on the street after nine years, and without exception they have reported that the habit of separation of incompatible foods has been continued ever since, and their whole families were observing the same precautions, simply because these men had been forced to observe the effects of this simple procedure on their own feelings and their own endurance during this four weeks of test.

Also, one, who had five arrows in his quiver, reported that

whereas most of his spare cash formerly went for doctor bills, now he never needed the doctor, as his wife and children, as well as himself, had been so well that there had been no necessity or excuse for calling his doctor.

This man also promoted himself, for his work was done so much better that his boss observed the change and gave him a better job, where he was able to make more money; for he was an employed man, one of the two who were not members of professional ranks.

In this group were two men who were suffering from opposite conditions, neither sick and neither well, the one sixty pounds over weight, the other fifteen pounds under weight.

The over weight man lost fifteen pounds and his endurance increased two hundred per cent; the other gained six pounds and his endurance increased one hundred and seventy-five per cent, yet both were doing the same things, merely separating their incompatible foods at each meal. And why should not this be the case, for both were away from the normal, and the body tended to go back to the normal, nothing more than this, and nothing less, merely a tendency toward the normal in both cases?

One of these men told me that he always fell asleep after his noon lunch. He was advised to change his noon meal to the morning, taking only milk and fruit for lunch, and this corrected the whole thing the very first day.

Fatigue is greatly aggravated by a heavy meal, immediately aggravated; and one of the best evidences of this is the afternoon siesta, that seems to follow the noon meal, if this has been heavy, and if the vitality is not very high; for it does sidetrack considerable vitality to initiate the digestion of a large meal, so with not a great deal of vitality on which to draw it is easily understood that the body requires some time to get this task under way; hence the desire to sleep after a meal, especially in the old or those failing in vitality.

If fatigue is so simple as this, why be tired, when it is wholly unnecessary? It is hard for people to believe that fatigue is really a self-controllable affair; but such is the case, of which the experiment before recited is sufficient proof.

Nor is this all; for the application of these same principles of feeding in many thousands of cases of varied type has shown uniformly the disappearance of fatigue, till after a year or two, in most cases, the sense of weariness is entirely gone, and physical endurance is present all the time, enabling one who is eating correctly to continue on hour after hour at work or play without seeming ever to tire.

The very same care necessary to prevent fatigue will also prevent the multitude of illnesses that make of life a sorry thing with so many people.

Remember that all disease, all fatigue, all old age, is this same accumulation of the acid end-products of digestion and metabolism, and you have the key to prevention of this trio of afflictions.

As the body loads up with this waste material it goes through stages, the first of which is pathological fatigue, the second disease of every type, the third is old age and the last and fourth stage is death, the end-point beyond which function ceases.

Sir William Arbuthnot Lane, the great London surgeon, said that there is but one disease; deficient drainage. This is true; for if we can eliminate fully every day all of these disease products, the acid end-products of digestion and meta· bolism, we remain without this accumulation that produces fatigue, disease, old age and death; in other words, we keep well, in normal funtion; while if these are allowed to accumu late we are candidates for all of these disasters.

Dr. George W. Crile, the eminent Cleveland surgeon, says that there is no natural death; that all deaths from so-called natural causes are the end-point of acid accumulation, the same statement as that of Sir Lane, and as right as the former statement; for there can be no natural death, if this is merely the end-point of a progressive acid saturation, and if this saturation is unnatural and unnecessary.

It is perhaps true that no one ever did so live as to wholly prevent these adventitious acids. To do so probably would require that we eat nothing at any time except wholly natural foods in their raw natural state, and these perhaps one at a time, and in no larger amount than strictly necessary for instant need.

It is not necessary that we be wholly normal, for we can approach this state near enough to be free from conscious fatigue, evident disease; we can defer the appearance of old age to far more distant times than we now think possible, and we can postpone the final accounting, the end-point of our tolerance, death, till such times as the mortician will become weary of waiting and perhaps go into some other business.

This is good, even if we do not achieve perfection; and to even approach it is to live far above the usual standard, and to enjoy the process of living as few mortals are given it to enjoy; also to achieve a plane in accomplishment that will make of our living something far above the crowd.

Is it worth while to make the attempt? Thousands who have made it have found the mode of life so superior to anything they have before experienced that few ever return to less scientific modes of living, but continue to make the eating of their daily foods a scientific study because they have found that this pays better dividends than anything they have before encountered.

During the next few years to come, any manner of living that will conserve energy, raise our efficiency, ease the burden of self-imposed fatigue, and at the same time cost nothing more than the ordinary habit of life, or even cost much less, if properly managed, will surely be a boon to the wage earner, as to everyone else; and the scientific selection and combination of foods will do all of these things for anyone who is a faithful adherent of the practice.

Fatigue is, in truth, the great American disease, the national handicap; and when we reflect that this condition is from the very same causes as all diseases of every sort, it gives us pause; for we are able to recognize the self-created character of both fatigue and disease.

If we put into the eradication of fatigue and disease the same amount of thought as we usually put into any successful line of business, we shall find that it pays much higher dividends than could any business, no matter how remunerative.

If we worry half as much about a decline in energy and endurance as we have been worrying about the decline in stocks, we shall find that we can control this leak a great deal easier than the drop in stocks.

If our finances are reduced to the vanishing point, and the cost of food is something more than incidental, then to know food values is to be in position to live on a few cents a day without the slightest loss in vitality and energy, and with little diminution in the pleasures of the table.

If the people of the United States had been rationed as closely during this panic (whatever this is) as was Denmark during the late war, we should have found that there was far more food available in the whole country than was needed, and no one need have gone hungry.

We eat wastefully every day; wastefully as to food, wastefully as to personal economy in the use of foods, wastefully in regard to our vitality, on the whole, wastefully of the greatest capital any nation or individual possesses—health and efficiency.

If waste is sinful, then we are a sinful people, for we are notoriously wasteful of food, even in times of financial stress;

[73]

and we waste more every day in this country than would have competently nourished all the starving poor of China, with those of several other nations included. Wastefulness of food has the commercial aspect on one side, and lowered efficiency on the other; and while the commercial waste is inexcusable, the waste of efficiency is unpardonable; for the facts of nutrition are available from laboratory records, and all that is needed is that these be taught to everyone in the whole ·land.

If we know someone is to be killed and do not warn him, we are guilty of his murder; accessories before the fact; and when we know that our friends, acquaintances, neighbors, are so living as to cause early decline and ultimately early death, and yet we do nothing to avert these two calamities, we are again accessories before a slow murder that is none the less sure than the revolver or the knife.

The facts of nutrition are available, if one will but read and study this fascinating subject. They do not require technical knowledge or training, for they are as simple as long division; and on account of their intimately personal interest to us, they should have more time devoted to their study than is usually thought necessary.

So often you will read in popular health columns the warning against monkeying with your food, avoiding the propaganda of the Health Faddist, coupled with the injunction to eat plenty of "good nourishing food;"—just the thing that everyone is doing and always has done; yet our country has more sickness than any other, with also the best food markets of the world. Any man who gives such directions is either ignorant himself of the facts of nutrition, or he is a paid propagandist of a far more dangerous type; one who does not dare to allow the public to know the simple facts of personal nutrition.

If he is the first he should be debarred from giving out dangerous information or misinformation; and if he is the second he should be banished to some country where wrong foods do not grow and cannot be obtained.

When our medical colleges teach the facts of nutrition as they now teach those of pathology, we shall soon begin to need fewer doctors, fewer nurses, fewer druggists, fewer morticians, and we shall have accumulated a huge potentiality of accomplishment in bounding health.

CHAPTER VI.

The Digestion of Food

IT is not how much we eat, but how much we can fully digest, absorb, metabolize, that counts, and also how fully we are able to scavenge the body of the resulting ashes, when we speak of nutrition.

To be well nourished is to take into the body everything it requires, to fully prepare and absorb this material, to metabolize or build it into the body or its stores of fuels, and to fully eliminate all the debris resulting from these processes.

A competently nourished body does not grow weary, it does not fall sick, it is at all times the faithful servant of the mind, it is able to accomplish everything physically possible to the human body. Nature intended us all to have such bodies, and but one thing has prevented this; our misinterpretation of nature's plain instructions.

The first step in the body's appropriation of food materials is their digestion, which is of importance in every consideration of health. Without competent digestion of our food we had much better omit it; for we will do far better wholly without food than to take this when unable to digest it properly.

Nature has given man a wonderful equipment for complete digestion or preparation of the foods eaten, and if we properly interpret the directions of nature we shall have gone far to digest fully all foods taken, preparing them for absorption. Without first digestion and absorption, metabolism, or the body's appropriation of the foods, could not occur, of course.

We think of the mouth as merely a sampling mill for the finer comminution and tasting of foods; but this is not all of its functions, for a very important step in digestion occurs in the mouth and can occur nowhere else. This is the splitting of the carbohydrate foods, the starches and sugars. For this purpose we are supplied with a little digestive ferment or hormone or

[76]

enzyme that we call ptyalin, whose duty it is to split the starches and sugars to lower forms before their entrance to the small intestine, where their further reduction occurs.

The stomach has no function in the digestion of starches and sugars except to act as a mixing chamber, thoroughly incorporating the saliva with its active ptyalin into the foods taken, and the starches and sugars thus thoroughly split into lower forms are ready for intestinal digestion. But (and here's the rub) this action can occur in nothing less than a positive alkalinity; the slightest acid reaction in the mass causing complete arrest of the splitting process, and even a neutral medium being sure to slow down and finally arrest this process of starchy reduction.

But you have always been taught that when we take food we produce gastric juice, one ingredient of which is hydrochloric acid.

This is perfectly true, but hydrochloric acid occurs in gastric juice just as the alkalies occur in the saliva, to activate the ferment that we call pepsin, whose function is the splitting of the protein, such as meats or eggs. If no protein is present when the starch enters the stomach the amount of hydrochloric acid is so small that it does not fully neutralize or overcome the alkalinity of the saliva present, except as we have habitually taken protein as a part of almost every meal for most of our lives, and we have in this way created a more or less fixed habit of acid production. For a time at first this acid habit persists, so it does make some difficulty in maintaining the necessary alkalin conditions for the continued splitting of the starches.

When we have followed correct eating for a considerable time this habit corrects itself, and we find that when starches are taken entirely separate from the proteins the amount of hydrochloric acid is negligible, as we are able to prove in the laboratory.

[77]

Now it must be evident that we are under necessity of maintaining the alkalinity for the splitting of the starches. Since the stomach cannot by any trick of legerdemain be both acid and alkalin at the same time, and as protein requires pepsin for its digestion, and as this ferment will not act except in a positive acidity, therefore it is asking too much of the stomach to take care of these two foods at the same time, the one requiring alkalinity for its digestion, the other acidity.

This is why we say that the simultaneous use of both concentrated starches and concentrated proteins is incompatible with complete digestion of either or both of these necessary and much abused and misunderstood foods.

Both are necessary to the body, both are mighty important, and we must have both, but not necessarily at the same time and in the same digestive task. So we take our starches and sugars at one meal, and our proteins at another, thus separating these two incompatible digestive tasks and allowing complete digestion of each separately.

Much has been said and written on this subject, and you will find eminent so-called scientists shouting from the housetops and from the pages of high class journals that this idea is the bunk, wholly bunk. All of which proves that they do not know, and should keep still till they have proved or disproved this simple thing.

When any man says this is unimportant to competent digestion he has already convicted himself of ignorance that is abysmal in the eyes of anyone who has tried it for even two weeks; for such knows that it does make a vast difference in one's feelings, in one's efficiency and freedom from fatigue, to separate these really incompatible tasks into two separate undertakings.

The argument is used that if this is wrong then nature herself made a serious mistake, for she combines in the grains ten per cent of protein with fifty per cent of starch, which is all true.

[78]

But the protein is here chiefly in the form of cellulose, an indigestible husk, and little food value is ever obtained from this, so it is quite unlikely that the stomach makes any effort to create an acid state for the activation of the pepsin for reduction of this protein.

Also, the cereal foods are so preponderently starchy that this type of digestion predominates over the acid type.

Meat is predominantly protein in character, so easily stimulates the production of the hydrochloric acid for the activation of the pepsin necessary to reduce the protein to lower forms; and the gastric juice during the digestion of meats or other forms of concentrated protein is high in hydrochloric acid, so there is active pepsin digestion.

If protein is present in foods to the extent of fifteen per cent we call this a protein food; or a legume, containing both protein and starch in proportions sufficient to class this as a mixture of both starch and protein in percentage sufficient to stimulate the ptyalin formation for the starchy digestion and the acid for the pepsin digestion of the protein, this is just why the mature legumes are not good, such as peas, beans, lentils, peanuts. It is difficult to digest these, unless they are immature, containing little of the starch with which they will predominate when fully developed.

Boston, with her baked beans, is also a sufferer from sour stomach two to three hours after the Saturday night feast; and Boston takes bicarbonate of soda for relief. Boston has tried to make the stomach take care of an alkalin task and an acid task at the same time, and it can't be done, in Boston or in Barbados.

The body has a wonderful adaptability to all sorts of conditions, but in keeping up this immunity to harmful practices it unnecessarily expends much needed energy, so suffers decline in vitality.

We cannot eat our cake and keep it, neither can we expend

vitality and at the same time conserve it. Vitality is life, function, accomplishment, continued youth, all of these things, and we cannot afford to expend it needlessly, thus shortening life, cutting down efficiency, interfering with enjoyment.

When food contains starch or sugar to the extent of twenty per cent this entitles it to classification as a concentrated carbohydrate, as potato, or banana. When this reaches fifty per cent, as in cereals or breads, then we have our highest concentration of unsplit starch.

So when we say starches and sugars should not be eaten with acids, or with protein that is going to stimulate acid formation, we are referring to concentrated carbohydrates, not to those below twenty per cent concentration.

In order to maintain the necessary alkalin stage for the digestion or reduction or conversion of the starches and sugars, we are under necessity of eliminating all acid or acid-compelling foods from the digestive tract. So when we eat bread we must see to it that we do not at the same time eat acid fruits or meats or eggs or fish or even cheese, all of these last requiring pepsin for their digestion, and the pepsin requiring hydrochloric acid for its activation.

If you have listened to the specious arguments of the "scientific" side of the discussion, then prove the thing for yourself, and you will be able to evaluate properly the arguments of those who have nothing but theory and so-called authority to offer. Facts have always discounted theory, and always will; so get the facts for yourself and let others be satisfied with unproved theory.

The writer is satisfied to let the whole subject of modern nutrition hang on this one proof, and if this proves correct, as it always will, then let the rest be accepted as corrollary facts.

If it were possible to get the foods eaten into the small intestine without this three or four hour residence in the stomach, we would never hear of the incompatibility of dissimilar foods; for when the food mass reaches the small intestine all digestion is carried on in an alkalin medium, all the intestinal ferments requiring alkalies to activate them. The saliva with its ptyalin initiates starch digestion, if the medium is kept alkalin; not otherwise. The gastric juice with its pepsin initiates protein digestion, if the medium is acid; not otherwise.

It would seem that no further argument is necessary to indicate the incompatibility of the digestion of starches and proteins at one and the same time, but if further argument seems necessary, then try it out for yourself and on yourself, and note the results. Two weeks should be enough to convince anyone, but if longer time is required, or seems to be desirable, then extend the period to four weeks, to make doubly sure.

After you have done this you will not be easily impressed with arguments against the wisdom of this separation, for you will then know first hand the truth of the real incompatibility of these dissimilar foods. If you will follow this practice long enough to lose your formed tolerance, you cannot go back to the practice of mixing proteins and starches without immediate notice from your stomach that you have made a serious mistake; one you will not likely repeat.

It is toleration that allows us to take increasing doses of even many irritant poisons without seeming harm; but never forget that this tolerance and seeming immunity to harmful effects is not natural, and is kept up at a very considerable expense in vitality continually.

The stomach retains the foods till they have reached a certain stage in their reduction, when the pylorus begins to open and the chyme, representing the partly digested contents, begins to filter out into the duodenum, the upper few inches of the small intestine, or jejunum; here the mass is alkalinized, if previously acid, for the intestinal juices are all strongly alkalin in character.

[81]

None of the intestinal ferments will function in anything less than a positively alkalin medium, so from here to the colon this alkalin state is maintained, else we could not digest our foods in the small intestine. Here all incompatibility ceases, and everything goes on harmoniously, for even the proteins require alkalin digestion from here on.

You will thus see that this is the most important step in the digestion of foods; for the stomach merely initiates the digestion of the protein, while the saliva initiates the digestion of the carbohydrates, the starches, and sugars. All the remainder of digestion of foods of every sort is up to the small intestine, which is able to carry on successfully only if the starches and proteins have each had the proper conditions higher up, in the mouth and stomach.

Digestion in the small intestine requires about six hours, as an average, when the mass begins to pass out into the colon, the sewer whose function it is to retain this chyme till absorption is finally completed to the point where little remains except the rubbish.

Fats and oils do not require any treatment to prepare them for action by the small intestine, as they are taken into this tube as fats or oils and there meet the bile in the duodenum and are emulsified and saponified, chiefly through the bile, and in this soapy form are absorbed directly into the blood stream by the lacteals.

Everything else absorbed from the small intestine goes through the circulation into the liver, there to submit to final inspection, when all nutritive material is allowed to pass into the general circulation, and the deleterious material is turned back again through the bile into the duodenum.

Thus the liver is a great filter that strains out of the blood brought to it the harmful material, unless we have created such a mass of this sort of material that in spite of the faithful old liver this gets by into the general circulation, as in migraine or "biliousness," and we go to the doctor "to get something for our torpid liver."

This is misjudging, even maligning, a faithful organ that is doing the very best it can with an impossible task. If you were a liver you would lie down on the job if you were half as badly treated, and you would feel injured were someone to apply a whip to make you work harder.

So instead of taking something to stimulate the liver, why not stop creating so much trouble and work for a very good organ?

No liver that is functioning as a liver should function when you are first born should ever give the slightest trouble later in life; and it would not if it were not for the fact that digestion is so miserably misunderstood and so imposed on that fermentations and putrefactions are forced on the digestive tract daily. The resulting debris is strained out so far as possible by an organ that is good enough for normal conditions but that may not be able to rise to impossible tasks.

When the food mass has been well digested, when absorption is well progressed, then the colon enters the picture; and here again is an organ that is good enough in everyone if given sane treatment, but that is not able always to contend with the putrid mass with which it is kept well filled in the average human animal.

When the simple laws of digestion have been flouted higher up in the digestive tract, the resulting fermentation and putrefaction is enough to stunt the activities of even a normally competent organ. And as this fails in function there is a vicious cycle developed, the poisonous character of the colon contents enervating or weakening the normally active muscular coat of the colon, thus interfering with its activity. As this activity slows down there is given more time for higher degrees of both fermentation and putrefaction to develop, till the higher this becomes the more is the colon poisoned, and the lower

[83]

sinks its function, till we see the hydraheaded monster of constipation rising up to plague us; and then again we make the mistake of whipping this tired horse because it is not keeping up with its work.

Verily, we are dunces when it comes to our treatment of our own bodies; for we are misinterpreting nature's plainest warnings and trying to avoid even seeing them, covering them up with the action of so-called remedies, instead of removing the cause of the whole foolish condition.

When any function begins to fail it is the custom of the physician as well as the wish of the patient that some stimulant for this lame function be given at once. If this be a failing endocrine gland the object is usually to supply this deficient function with that borrowed from some animal, usually the harmless sheep.

This is what we try to do in diabetes mellitus, for we recognize the evident failure of pancreatic function and inject into the subject the insulin obtained from the Langerhansian end of the pancreas of the sheep.

All our attempts to help failing function take the form of either a whip or a crutch, the one to stimulate function, the other to supplement it.

Neither plan is in any sense corrective, so never constructive, all a fussing with the end results of a condition the cause of which is either wholly misunderstood or totally ignored.

There is some reason why the function of any organ fails, whether a ductless gland, a viscus, or a secretory function; and instead of recognizing the primary or predisposing cause, the usual custom is to do something for the condition as it presents, not constructive, and far too often destructive.

If your neighbor develops lameness, say arthritis, and he refuses to suffer the pain necessary to maintain motion, you are not doing him any constructive good when you hand him a crutch or a wheel chair; you are only recognizing his difficulty in walking and trying to do something for the symptom.

It is even so with all our medical treatment for disease; for all we try to do is to stimulate or assist or supplement some function in disrepair, without doing anything to correct the underlying conditions that have seemed to make this assistance necessary.

If the continued function of an arthritic joint depends on daily use of the painful limb, then the introduction of crutch or wheel chair becomes destructive, as it defeats the attempt to return to normal; and too often the victim resigns himself to the wheel chair and thus fails to regain the function of the painful member; a destructive procedure. It is even so with our ductless gland deficiencies; for if we continually supply their function vicariously they cease to develop their usual function, and this will be destroyed by disuse. How often we see the victim of the pepsin or hydrochloric acid habit drift into chronic dyspepsia, or apeptic or achlorhydric state, through supplying these necessities for protein digestion vicariously for too long a time!

The writer sees many of these cases totally lacking in protein digestion without these artificial aids; yet every one of these will in time develop again a normal amount of both pepsin and hydrochloric acid if fed naturally for several months.

During these past twenty-six years of the natural treatment of disease he has never found it necessary to introduce one dose of either pepsin or hydrochloric acid, recognizing the fact that protein digestion has broken down, yet refusing to believe that because the body cannot take care of protein normally that therefore we must MAKE it do so by introduction of these supposed aids to this broken-down digestion. It is much more natural to withhold this type of foods, especially as they are not necessary through rather long periods of time, till nature again supplies the missing ferment and its activator, which nature will never fail to do if given a fair chance.

This is constructive treatment, though doing nothing at all, for it has allowed nature to rebuild a function badly out of repair, but not irreparable. In very truth the most constructive form of treatment is very often the doing of nothing at all till nature has time and opportunity to recreate the missing function.

Separate your incompatibles and eat natural foods.

CHAPTER VII.

Normal Alkalinity

THE whole medical profession is up against the fact that all of our standards are estimated on averages, for we have no way to arrive at a normal standard, failing to find in this whole world a normal individual.

The average man is very far from the normal, even that man who has been living quite closely to the rules of nutrition that are now known to conserve vitality most; for we start with imperfect heredity and build on this, year by year, a toxic state that tends to grow deeper with each year of life.

If heredity is ideal, if from birth we are fed exactly right, if we have taken sufficient exercise to thoroughly oxidize our waste, if we have slept sufficiently in normal surroundings, and if we have eaten nothing habitually that in any way tends to lower our alkalin reserve, then we should present a normal or near normal condition; then only would we be safe as standards for others.

The haziest of ideas prevail as to the normal alkalinity of the human blood stream; and while it is not possible to arrive at this exactly, having no normal standards, yet those patients who for several years have been building up an alkalin reserve, through the 80/20 idea of relative acid-alkali balance, when they present for a pH estimation of blood alkalinity, are told uniformly that they are suffering from an alkalosis, or too high ratio of alkali to acid.

From the standpoint of averages a pH 7.5 is an alkalosis; yet when the alkalinity of the blood is sufficiently high to show a 7.5 pH there is extremely high functional activity, with comparable feeling of good health, mental activity and physical efficiency.

Most observers believe that a pH of 7.1 to 7.3 is within

the normal limits, again demonstrating that they have always dealt with the average, not the normal.

Normals should not be much if any below pH 7.5, judging by the averages of those who have conserved their alkalin reserve for several years, through proper ratio of base-forming foods to the acid-forming kinds.

It may seem strange that the slight difference between a pH 7.1 and 7.6 spells the wide difference between an acidosis and an alkalosis; yet this is true; and even this slight variation makes all the difference between function of the most chaotic variety and that of high efficiency.

We told you earlier that the function of every organ and tissue depends on the height, breadth and depth of the alkalin reserve; and the lower this is the lower the function; and, conversely, the higher this alkalin reserve the higher the degree of functional activity.

To maintain this high alkalinity of the body fluids is to eat in such a way that the alkalin or base-forming foods must predominate over the acid-forming foods in an 80/20 ratio, eighty per cent of the daily intake being of the base-forming, and not more than twenty per cent of the acid-forming varieties.

We speak loosely of an acidosis, which would mean, literally, an acid state of the body, a thing clearly impossible, for function will suspend at once in the presence of even a 50/50 ratio of these two opposites, and this means death; for death is merely the suspension of all function, the end-point beyond which the body is unable to carry on.

So we are under compulsion to keep up an alkalin reserve at all times sufficient to maintain function. If this reserve is low, the function of all kinds will correspond; and if high, then also will function be high; and function is life.

Function is normal, as we see the normal, when the pH of the blood is at a pH 7.5; but at this high level the case is so rare that the observer at once calls it an alkalosis, and seeks to create a higher acid state by use of much meat or other acid-forming foods.

After eating, the pH will undergo change, depending chiefly on the character of foods taken, those leaving behind an alkalin ash tending to raise the pH, and those leaving behind an acid ash tending in the opposite direction, naturally.

The best time for a pH estimation is first thing in the morning, when the body has completed digestion and largely also absorption, also when metabolism is at its height and the debris of the day before very largely eliminated. Then we get a true picture of the body alkalinity, uninfluenced by foods.

If you will keep continually in mind that in no other way than through daily dietary habit can we build up and conserve an alkalin reserve, then you will be impressed with the necessity of seeing that each day's intake shall contain plenty of the alkalin or base-forming foods, and not too much of the acid-forming foods, the convenient ratio being 80/20, or four times as much food taken every day that will leave behind an alkalin ash as of the foods that will leave behind an acid ash.

It is true that by taking in alkalin drugs, minerals of alkalin character, we can temporarily raise the alkalin reserve, but these mineral alkalies are no part of the body, as they must be taken in the colloidal state to be of use permanently in function.

These minerals tend to deposit in the body, acting as foreign matter, and many of them are difficult of elimination, so tend to accumulate in the tissues, upsetting the normal acid-alkali balance. It is only in this way that we can create an alkalosis, except in those conditions of degenerative change, as cancer, where the disintegration of the mass throws into the system quantities of alkalin debris.

A noted cancer researcher not long ago told the writer that he had taken the pH of blood entering the cancer area and again leaving this field, and found uniformly the pH of that returning from the cancer higher than that entering it, the reverse of the normal, for the body picks up its acids from the tissues, through oxidation of fuels there, or the death of body tissue, and the venous blood is charged with these acid end-products to be carried to the lungs and there eleminated as carbon dioxide and water.

Alkalosis and cancer are twins, for cancer always throws into the circulation vast quantities of alkalin debris, creating an alkalosis. This has led to the erroneous idea that a too high degree of alkalinity predisposes to cancer; yet I am sure you will see that the alkalin condition is the result, and not the cause.

Cancer never develops in normal tissues, those nourished with a proper blood supply; and this means a higher degree of alkalinity than is thought to be normal, judging by the usual standards of low alkalinity that are presented by the average case in any condition of health or disease.

We too often confuse effects with causes, which is not surprising when we consider that all our medical studies have been directed toward pathology, the evidence of disease, not its cause.

In the past, money has been spent like water in so-called cancer research, all of this wasted utterly; for the studies were of cancer, not the pre-cancer states of the blood, which is the only field of study that will ever lead to the discovery of why some cases develop cancer and others do not.

The experimental creation or transplantation of cancers in the laboratory animals, usually mice or white rats, does not help in the least our understanding of the predisposing conditions to cancer formation in the human. Only in the past ten years has there seemed to be any tendency to study pre-cancer states of the blood, or early states of the blood in cancer incidence.

From now on there will be more study directed toward these blood conditions in early cancer than the actual conditions in late cancer states; but we shall have to go farther than this, keeping record of blood alkalinity in numerous cases before there is any evidence of malignancy. Then, in the cases where this later develops, a careful study of blood conditions earlier can be compared with conditions after the malignancy has developed, a form of study that may require one or more generations to complete to anything like a definite proof.

However, we should be frank enough to admit that up to the very present time we have gotten nowhere in cancer research. Evidently we have been on the wrong track so far, and we should be willing to try an entirely different one.

If the blood shows a picture higher than pH 7.5 we are at once suspicious that already a malignant growth is present, for such high tests of alkalinity are rare indeed in other than cancer states.

It is thinkable that in one whose daily dietary is wholly of vegetables and fruits this pH might be even higher without suspicion of malignancy, as in this case there would be left behind such quantities of alkalies that it would be suspicious indeed, when we think of the average blood picture.

The alkalin foods are colloidal in structure, as against mineral in such alkalin minerals as soda or magnesia. In the colloidal state these do not tend to accumulate in the system, but readily oxidize and pass out through the ordinary channels of elimination, leaving again the normal ratio or the normal pH.

The mineral alkalies through their difficult oxidation and elimination tend to pile up in the body, creating an alkalosis for the time being, or till the blood can again eliminate the excess.

Many a case of ordinary sour stomach has used common baking soda, or sodium bicarbonate, for many years, and always there is sour stomach if the soda is omitted.

These mineral alkalies tend to neutralize acids with which they come in contact, but do nothing to limit acid formation, so are not curative of the hyperacid condition.

[91]

So long as the soda habit persists just so long will the sour stomach persist, as every user well knows.

Stop the soda but correct the incompatibilities in the daily intake, and no soda will be necessary.

Many of these cases of chronic sour stomach have never had one day of this after completely separating these incompatible foods; which means that when either starch or sugar in concentrated form is eaten, then no acids and no protein, such as meats or eggs, is taken at the same time.

This is stomach acidity, a matter of digestion and its interruption, and has nothing to do with body acidity or its opposite, alkalosis.

When the pH of the blood or body fluids is at 7.5 it means that there is a very considerable alkalin reserve available with which to tie up or bind the adventitious acids as these form.

This is what we mean by an alkalin reserve. Even though the difference between an acidosis and an alkalosis is very slight, measured in terms of pH, yet this difference is most vital to health; for with much alkali available for union with the acids as they form there is no acid effect; while with little available free alkali the acids find not enough alkali to bind them fully, and then we get the acid effects that we call acidosis.

Starvation is an acidosis, for with the intake of base-forming food withheld from the digestive tract there is nothing with which to tie or bind the acids, and we get the acid effects as a very prominent condition in starvation.

During the fast the body continues to give off its acids of decomposition, as the body cells die and give up their acid debris to the circulation. So it is easy to understand that the fasting body continues to exhibit the evidences of acidosis till the very end of the fast; but when base forming foods are taken these acid symptoms disappear very quickly.

The fast is a good thing for the body, as it offers opportunity to unload without at the same time loading up.

[92]

During the progress of a fast, when no food of any kind is taken, the alkalin reserve may be kept up nicely by the intake of considerable amounts of any unsweetened fruit juice, together with two or three ounces daily of fresh vegetable juice.

While the acid fruit juices might be thought contra-indicated in acid states this is not the case; for, while they do contain citric, malic, or tartaric acids, these are easily volatilizable substances, and it is safe to say that within an hour after the taking of an unsweetened fruit juice the body does not contain one grain of the acid taken.

With these acids are bound up in the fresh fruits common alkalies, such as lime, soda, and potash, generally in the form of phosphates, the very best and most needed of all the alkalies required by the body.

As the salts are broken up in the digestive tract, the acid is driven out of combination with the alkalies and exhaled from the lungs. Although some of these salts find their way out through the skin, and slightly also through the urinary tract and bowel, yet chiefly through breathing do we get rid of the acids of fresh fruits.

Their alkalies released from the combination with acids are deposited in the system, adding to our alkalin reserve, for these are all colloidal in form, not minerals, so they reinforce the alkalin reserve of the body as nothing else will do.

The salts of the fresh vegetable juice are also strongly alkalin, and these, together with the alkalin salts from the fruits, very competently reinforce the alkalies of the body; and fasting with these fresh juices has all the advantages of the absolute fast with none of the disadvantages.

When no solid food is taken, no addition to the calories of the body, the effect is the same as that of the absolute fast.

When undertaking the fast it is well to take every day one to three quarts of fresh orange juice, fresh apple cider, or fresh grape juice, always without sugar; and to each glass of

[93]

the fruit juice add a tablespoonful or more of the fresh vegetable juice.

Vegetable mills, or vegetable juice extractors may be had, or one can grind the vegetables in an ordinary food chopper, using a rather fine knife, and press the juices out through a potato ricer or other form of press. This fresh juice may be set in the ice-box for as much as a week without danger of spoiling.

The best vegetables to use for this purpose are carrots, turnips, beets, of the root vegetables, and all sorts of top vegetables, such as spinach, beet tops, chard, celery, onion tops, watercress, broccoli, or any green vegetable that contains juice.

These with the fruit juices are excellent for neutralizing an acid state, whether during the fast or not, and taken without food they have even more effect.

Many a case of acute illness has been given up to die and has been brought back to safety by use of these simple juices, with all food of every sort interdicted, till recovery was well on the way and the patient again expressed a desire for food.

Of all the insane practices to which the poor deluded invalid has submitted through all the ages past, the most insane, the most inexcusable, is feeding during illness, feeding anything at all except the simple juices that require practically no digestion and that leave behind nothing but alkalies of which the body stands in need.

During sickness of any kind the body is exhibiting an acute acid state, for this is just what illness is. To add to this by the further intake of so much acid-forming material as is represented by the ordinary invalid's diet is surely pouring oil on fire; and when the ill recover under this form of mistreatment it is in spite of this, never because of it.

It is mighty hard to kill some people, and they do get well in spite of the craziest forms of treatment; but remember, this is never because of the treatment, but really in spite of it.

When you hear anyone say that acidosis is a greatly over-discussed condition, and that very little attention should be paid to it, you will know that such a one has never looked into the thing, or practiced medicine along the lines of detoxication, therefore knows nothing of the effect of acid and how easily this is obviated.

Years ago Alexander Haig, an eminent Scottish physician, gave to the medical world a discussion of uric acid that had them all trying his theories; and for a long time uric acid held the boards.

Haig's idea was much too limited, for he ascribed to uric acid the entire role of body acidifier, when as a matter of fact it is but one of many, and, except in free meat eaters who take little exercise, uric acid is by no means even the commonest of the systemic acids that make so much trouble in reducing body alkalinity.

Like every other partial truth it made a ripple of excitement for a time, and like every other ripple it was gradually lost to sight and forgotten.

Truth never dies; and Haig's uric acid theory still lives; but its unimportance caused it to fall into disuse for a long time.

It contained enough truth, however, to keep it before the minds of the one per cent of thinking physicians; and as our chemistry has so broadened during the past twenty-five years of experimental laboratory studies in nutrition, a much broader conception of acids as a cause of disease is coming to be realized, though the dietary causes of this state never have been understood by the mass of even this elect one per cent of physicians who can think independently and reason correctly from cause to effect.

When that time comes, if it ever does come, when the causes of disease are understood to be simply an accumulation of the acid end-products of digestion and metabolism in a body unable to eliminate these as fast as they are created, then indeed will the human race begin to be delivered from so much infernal experimentation and guesswork; and then will the huge mortality from both medical and surgical practice sink to almost the vanishing point.

Then the expensive diagnostic clinic will fade away as snow in the hot regions; for the matter of diagnosis will cease to be of paramount interest or importance, and the thing necessary will be an estimation of the extent of accumulation of acid debris, and the distance the body has already departed from normal vitality and resistance.

Then it will not be necessary for the asthmatic or the tubercular victim to seek higher and drier climates; for recovery will then be a question of proper, thorough, and deep detoxication, and such dietary correction as will limit the formation of the deleterious acid end-products to that resulting from body change and body activity.

That it is possible to so arrange the food intake daily as to limit this formation of debris from food to practically zero, is a matter that does not need demonstration, for it has been amply demonstrated in many thousands of cases not found in the data of the practitioner of medicine or surgery of the classical sort, but rather in the records of the physiological laboratories working with the feeding of the laboratory animals, and in the unofficial records of those few physicians who have been applying clinically for years these very same laboratory findings.

It is one thing to reach certain fundamental conclusions in laboratory studies of the animal, and still another thing to prove clinically on the human the ultimate truth of the theories born from laboratory research in the nutritional field. Both records are replete with abundant proof of the before-stated fact that we, all of us, animals and the human, are merely a composite of what we eat, daily, yearly and as a life habit. If you do not agree with this statement then it is again pertinent to inquire, of what is one made?

The alkalin reserve can be maintained only through use of base-forming foods and proper combinations of these.

CHAPTER VIII.

The Public Feeding Trough

THE number of those who are compelled to depend on the public eating place is beyond doubt very large.

This includes school life away from home, and business life under employment conditions; and while it is not easy to adhere to any feeding schedule that is radically different from the commonly accepted standards, yet this is possible, and becomes increasingly easy as one adheres to the proper plan rigidly.

Do not blame the hotel or restaurant when you cannot get your foods in proper form or proper combination, as public eating habits are a creation of the public itself, and every caterer to the public seeks to meet the usual demand in variety and form.

In fact the success of any public eating place depends very largely on how closely it interprets the public demand and adheres to public habit.

When common habit changes, so will the bill-of-fare change, and not till then; for those purveyors of food that have sought to educate the public into proper habits, without exception, have found that this public did not wish to be educated.

Such altruistic attempts have brought nothing but failure, and are bound to fail till a sufficient number are educated in better eating habit to create a demand for proper food, properly combined, and properly served.

Already in certain cities there is a sufficient number of such educated eaters to supply customers in numbers that will maintain a modest patronage for such institution as knows how to cater to this one branch of scientific eaters—those who place results before the momentary pleasure of the table, and who eat for a purpose.

While it is important to eat those foods that the body requires every day, it is also important that these foods should be thoroughly enjoyed; for food taken without appetite or enjoyment is of little use to a body that knows what it wants when it wants it.

If we are free from erroneous habit in selecting and combining food, we may rely absolutely on appetite to tell us when to eat, what to eat, and how; but almost from birth we have built up habit in food selection that rules us afterward throughout life; so these primal instincts in food selection have become notoriously unreliable. To get back to normal habit is to smash present habit for a time.

There is a very potent way to accomplish this, though many may think it a ruthless and harsh way. This is to stop eating everything till the appetites all leave, as they will in a few days, and then begin to select the food according to need instead of desire. After doing this for a few weeks it will be discovered that the new habit brings more pleasure in eating than the old hit-or-miss habit.

If one wishes to change the appetite quickly, the shortest and by far the best method is to take three heaping tablespoonfuls of Epsom or Glauber salts dissolved in a half pint of water first thing in the morning, while the stomach is entirely empty, or take a half pint of concentrated Pluto water, which is a mixture of both these salts, and confine the entire intake of nourishment to fruit juices unsweetened.

Continue this for about three days, and you will find that your interest in foods has folded its tent and stolen away, and then you will be in position to build up any form of habit you please.

Eating habit is subject to change, but unless the necessity for this change is thrust upon one it is seldom made, for we tend always to fall into habit. As it is easier to continue any daily habit than to make a stand against it and ruthlessly break it, you will find that but few people make any attempt whatever to change their usual custom in any particular, chiefly so in regard to their eating.

It becomes of extreme importance that very early in life proper eating habit should be inculcated; for we are such creatures of habit that after we have done any certain thing in some certain way for a few times we tend to continue to do this thing in the same way ages on end.

The principles of food incompatibility can be taught to children no more than three or four years of age, as I have witnessed many times; and these little children are then saved for life against wrong combination of their daily foods. I have seen such little ones sit at table and correct the combination mistakes of the older members of the family who knew better, but who had formed the habit of taking certain incompatible foods, and who did not feel well till this error had been committed.

By the time children have reached school age their eating habits are quite fixed, and it is important that they should be fixed right as early as possible, for every year that wrong habit persists it is increasingly difficult to make radical changes in this.

In growing children the matter of first importance is that they get every day everything of which the body stands in need; and it is of scarcely less importance that these things be so combined as to prevent the chaotic chemistry that is created from wrong combinations of food.

If all children were properly trained in combination of dissimilar or similar foods, the next generation would not suffer from public eating habits, for you would find these changing just as the demand changed.

It is too much to expect the caterer to the public eating habit to experiment in education of his patrons, for he knows well that they will go elsewhere to eat if he does not give them the things they most wish to have, whether right or wrong.

The usual understanding of proper dietary habit is to eat

the good, plain, everyday foods that are so common, and to avoid pastries, fancy dishes, and condiments. There is no faster way to wreck the human machine than to subsist continually on meats, white breads, boiled potatoes, perhaps pie, with coffee sweetened with white sugar; yet this probably would be called a good wholesome meal.

The introduction of certain raw foods, as vegetable salads and fresh fruits, is all that keeps such a diet as this from producing deficiencies that are sure to cut down health and performance; and it is this little leaven that leavens the whole lump, else we would not be here.

Analyze the hotel meal, or any public table d'hote menu, and you will find it built about this very combination of foods, and too often a small amount of raw food, limited to a lettuce leaf with two or three slices of tomato or cucumber, a gesture that is too often unnoticed by the diner.

A proper salad, one that well fills a salad plate, would do much to take the curse off the usual meal, but this should be eaten first, to make sure it is enjoyed. Then if the diner will drink a glass or two of milk and take some raw fruit unsweetened for dessert, he will save much acid formation, and at the same time do much to build up his present depleted alkalin reserve.

The laborer at physical work, or the athlete in training, needs a great deal more of the fuel variety of foods than does the sedentary subject. Breads, potatoes, starches, sugars, may be consumed in much larger quantity by the active than the inactive, of course. But no matter what he needs, these can safely be met without disregard of the unchangeable laws of chemistry that tell us that the stomach cannot at the same time maintain an alkalin state for the digestion of starches, and produce an acid state for the digestion of meats. The only reason we are not immediately poisoned painfully by such mixtures is that for so long we have made this mistake that the body has built up a tolerance that enables us to carry on in spite of this error, in semblance of the normal.

Stop eating together the incompatible foods for a few weeks or a very few months and then try to return to this and see what happens.

A young man recently out of college and the athletic squad, who had very creditable performances to his record, degenerated into a bond salesman, and almost wholly to the desk part of the business.

His former athletic appetite, coupled with a nearly sedentary habit, soon produced the usual effects of rapid intoxication; so that by the time he presented himself for treatment he was suffering from the usual acid stomach, indigestion, gas, and constipation, with what he called biliousness and sick headache.

His dietary habit was corrected and he was taught the necessity for keeping the colon emptied every day. For two or three months he gloried in his return to athletic condition, and his bond sales picked up wonderfully as a natural result.

His convivial habits led to contacts with many bibulous friends who believed in eating everything in sight, and he became dissatisfied with his necessity for so much thought in selecting and combining his foods. He asked complainingly how much longer he would have to continue this care, and was told just so long as he wished to be well. He asked if it would do him any serious harm if he broke training for one night and ate anything he pleased in any combination that happened, and was told to try it.

Two days later he presented himself penitently with the report of his experiment, saying he was never so sick in his life as he had been for a whole day after his lapse, and promised that he would never repeat this experiment; and it is doubtful whether he will.

During perhaps three months he had experienced freedom from the usual acid accumulations that had before been his daily handicap, and during this rather short period he had lost much of his former tolerance for acids of fermentation, so he was cheerfully told to try it, as a trial after even three months of rather strict regime would surely be enough to convince him that he could not again go back to heterogeneous mixtures of incompatible foods without suffering at once.

We all carry this tolerance for incompatible foods, but at a very considerable sacrifice in vitality that should be available for daily performance, rather than being tied up in the form of a cultivated tolerance.

When the body has available all of its vitality, without being under necessity of tying up so much of this to maintain a tolerance for adventitious acids, then performance is on a much higher plane, both the physical and the mental, as experience with the plan has definitely taught through application to thousands of cases of every type during the past twenty-six years of assiduous adaptation.

Again, we cannot eat our cake and keep it, and we cannot tie up vitality and at the same time have the full amount available for any emergency that might arise.

Life, vitality, health, are synonyms for alkalinity; and when the alkalin reserve is up to full quota or nearly, then we have all of these things; and they shrink in exactly the ratio in which the reserve of free alkali declines.

Thus you see the necessity for the intake of much alkalin or base-forming food each day, and the equal necessity for holding down to small proportions the acid-forming material, which leads to the 80/20 standard before mentioned.

It is not possible at anything less than a well appointed hotel or restaurant to get the amount of vegetables and fruits desired for easy approach to this ratio; but one can at least stress the vegetables and fruits more, and the meats and starches less; and always one can separate his foods into compatible groups by an understanding of what constitutes a concentrated carbohydrate food and what a concentrated protein.

The concentrated carbohydrate foods are breads, cereals,

all products of grains, starchy roots or extracts from roots, such as tapioca and sago, also all sugars and very sweet things of every kind.

The protein group comprises meats, eggs, fish, cheese; and the meats include every form of flesh food, no less chicken or lamb than beef or pork, for all have about this same ratio, 18% protein, or nearly.

Fish include every variety of shell fish, as well as the vertebrate varieties; and of all the group the innocent oyster is highest in acid-forming potentiality.

Never forget that the carbohydrate group requires alkalin conditions for complete digestion, and that the protein group requires acid conditions for stomach digestion; so when these two opposite types of food are found in the stomach at the same time, chaos of digestion results. We are not conscious of this fact because we have habituated ourselves to this habit of combination always, and only the Lord knows how much of vitality or how much of accomplishment and enjoyment we have sacrificed.

We can realize something of what this has cost us by desisting from the mistake for a few weeks and observing the effect, then by a long enough continuance of the correct habit of combination for two or three or more months, till we have lost much of our tolerance for the effects, and then by an attempted return to the wrong habit of combination.

In any hotel we can take our meats or other form of protein at one meal, and our carbohydrates, such as bread, at another, thus separating the two dissimilar tasks widely, and so escaping this one great cause of acid-formation.

We can do this in our own home, at the tables of our friends, any place where food is served, and without the necessity for an à la carte service, simply by leaving out the incompatible articles.

If we elect to make the meal starchy, then we can have all the bread we wish, all the vegetables, all the raw salads, if we

[103]

dress these without acid, and all the sweet fruits or ice cream or other unrefined sweet desert.

If we prefer to make the meal a protein type, then we take the meat or other protein, the vegetables, raw salads, dressing these with acid, as lemon juice and oil, and also we can have all the acid fruit we desire as dessert.

If we take the starchy type, then we leave out all the acids and all the proteins that will produce a hydrochloric acid in the stomach, thus preserving the alkalin conditions necessary for the digestion of the starches.

If we take the protein type, then we leave out all the starchy and sweet things.

If we must have our coffee we may sweeten this when accompanying a starchy type meal, but we must abjure the sugar when taking a protein meal.

All very simple, isn't it? When you first try to apply it, however, it will not seem so simple; for if there is any one subject that is little understood among average people it is this subject of foods and what they do to us.

Do not make the excuse that because you are compelled to eat at public eating houses therefore diet in any form is impossible to you.

A certain amount of care will bear fruit anywhere on the face of the earth; for there is food everywhere, if man can live at all in the surroundings.

Patients who are devotees of proper eating, and who have travelled much, report that everywhere they were able to stick to compatible eating, but not everywhere were they able to get the foods in as vital form as they could desire.

When the digestion is weak it is usual to find directions to take only the "bland" foods, meaning by this the soft foods that are not hard to digest. A soft diet as usually interpreted, will ruin anyone completely if followed long enough, for it is wholly a devitalized diet.

[104]

Nature does not create much of man's food in bland form, except the banana and a very few others.

Nature gives us teeth sufficient for us to prepare for digestion every type of food that is good for us; and while it is possible to properly nourish oneself without teeth, it is at the same time much easier if we have these aids to the preparation of our foods.

Those without teeth, the edentulous victims, have to be satisfied with those foods that do not require thorough chewing; such as "pap," mushy cereals, milk, soft fruits, puréed vegetables, soups, all of which are competent for every need if the selection is right and if the combination does not violate chemical laws.

O'Leary, the walker, at an age when most men have ceased athletic struggle, will walk around the bases twice while any speedy man selected by the team travels three times around the same base paths.

This means that O'Leary travels two hundred and forty yards while the ball player runs three hundred and sixty yards, but O'Leary does the distance heel-and-toe, while the ball player runs at top speed.

O'Leary is practically without teeth, so is forced to eat only soft foods; yet at a good age he is athletic and has great endurance.

He eats breads, which surely must be whole grain breads, but he "dunks" these in his coffee. 1 am not sure whether he uses cream or sugar or both in the coffee, but it is presumable that he uses both, as his expenditure of energy in these walks would call for much creation of caloric stores, such as would be furnished by the starchy bread and also the sugar and cream.

If you wish to lose your teeth early quit chewing hard foods; for nature will not long perpetuate a useless function, and when the teeth cease to be needed they will soon depart.

This is not the entire reason, however, for the usual deficient dietary gives us little material with which to make good the materials of which the teeth are constructed.

Foods poor in lime and silicates will not support teeth, even if these are given proper work; but a combination of complete foods and foods hard enough to compel thorough mastication will insure perfect teeth not occasionally, but always.

In selecting starches, if one will always adhere to those containing all of their original ingredients, instead of those of refined character, much material that will reinforce the teeth will be included; for refined flours are one of the greatest causes of decay of teeth, as also the refined sugars.

The lime and silicates and fluorides so necessary for the teeth are missing in the refined flours, while the bran and pericarp contain these things; so when at a hotel table always ask for whole wheat, rye or graham bread, to make sure to get these very necessary chemicals. When the majority of the patrons of public eating houses demand the dark breads these will appear on every table, just as the demand for everything must precede this thing in the market.

So, do not blame public eating houses for the public eating habit; rather blame the public eating habit for the condition of the public eating place.

If the whole grain breads were chiefly in evidence, if the vegetables were cooked conservatively, if raw salads occurred in ample amounts, rather than table decorations, and if the incompatibilities of every meal were known and respected, there would never be cause for complaint against the public feeding trough; for every such place is a reflection of the trend of ordering in vogue.

Just as every dealer seeks to keep on display the things that his customers are most apt to desire, just so will the hotels seek to feature the things most often called for; and the hotel will always reflect the desires of its patrons.

This puts it up to the eater himself to correct the habit of the public eating house; and only he can do the job.

CHAPTER IX.

Fear

AND what has fear to do with health? Fear is both a cause and a result of disease. Fear per se will paralyze all function, if deep enough. It is just as true that disease will cause fear, and thus a vicious cycle develops.

As a cause of disease fear is a purely psychic affair, fear from any cause being a hindrance to normal function. As a result of disease fear is one of the most frequent, as disease of any sort, whether slight or severe, reacts to produce fear of consequences.

The most frequent source of fear every day is the personal health, giving rise to more forebodings, more depressing anticipations, than any other thing, even the stock market during a slump.

Many people, otherwise good and sensible, spend their precious vitality very lavishly in worrying over their health, or its lack.

To a physician who has for forty-two years listened to the minute details furnished by most patients, there remains little doubt that the thoughts of disease and aberrations of health occupy too large a place by far in the thinking of the average person.

Fear hangs over the head of so many people continually that life is not very alluring; and yet, however discouraging the outlook, few are willing to separate themselves from living. The fear that life may terminate soon, or that lingering disease is just around the corner, has spoiled many a life that might otherwise have been pleasant and profitable to the sufferer and friends.

Fear is bred directly from misunderstanding of things as they are, and what we do not understand we are quite apt to fear most.

[107]

So often a lion in the path is found to be merely a moss-covered stone, and a huge serpent nothing more than a crooked limb of a fallen tree.

"I am an old man, and have seen much trouble, most of which never happened."

If all the things we anticipate with dread and fear were to have happened to us, great would have been our calamity; but it is safe to say that not one per cent of anticipated danger actually materializes.

So that ninety-nine per cent of our anticipatory fears were groundless, and nothing we did or could do would have changed the conditions, for there was nothing to fear, and nothing developed; and the one per cent is never helped in the slightest degree by fears, so the entire 100 per cent of worry is foolish. We waste too much vitality needlessly in this way.

If you think fear is not a large factor in health then your observation of the effects of fear has been very limited.

It can be demonstrated in the laboratory, with the x-ray, that fear actually paralyzes peristalsis of the intestine, meaning that the worm-like movements of the intestine, those traveling circles of compression by which the bowel passes its contents on toward the exit, are completely interdicted during acute fear; as in the well known case of the cat when a dog barks nearby.

In the case of the cat it was two hours afterward before peristalsis had resumed its normal rate and rhythm. If fear will do this to a cat then it will do the same thing to a man; for the intestine is subject to brain control, just as is every other function of the body.

If fear of acute and intense variety will paralyze the sympathetic control, then fears of lesser degree will partially inhibit the sympathetic, thus lowering the function of every organ supplied by the nerves; and all organs are so supplied.

Fear will blanch the cheek instantly, and it will blanch the hair in one night, as has been observed so often in fright.

If this emotion has such immediate effect, is it not fair to suppose that accumulated fears of lesser degree will have a cumulative effect in interfering with all function?

Some people, especially some women, live in a state of perpetual fear; and such are never healthy. It is said in extenuation: "The poor woman is not well."

This has been true always so far as I have been able to observe; and not only will no one be subject to such a state of fear if well, but it is equally true that no one who harbors fear can be well.

The two things are complementary, each the cause as well as effect of the other, representing one of the most pointed examples of the vicious cycle.

Now if fear is in any degree the result of the lack of normal function, or health, and if this lack of health is self-created from well defined causes that are easily controllable, then why in the name of all that is sane should anyone ever worry about his or her health? If you knew for a fact that you may be sick or well just as you obey certain laws or fail to observe them, would you then worry about your health? Of course not, for then there would be nothing to worry about.

You would need to decide whether your health is worth the pains required to observe the laws, or whether it is not; and the choice would be yours and the result just what you would deserve.

It was remarked shortly before this that we fear what we do not understand. This is exemplified beautifully in our fears of diseases; for if we understood this as we should, there would not be one thing to worry about, for we could be well or ill, as we chose.

It is perfectly true that if we understood what causes disease we would be shorn of every excuse for worry about our health, for we could not with any semblance of excuse worry about something that we can control. It is so evident that we think we cannot control disease, or we would not worry about it, that the worry itself is proof enough that we have no fundamental understanding of our own body processes in either health or disease. Worry is nothing but fear, and fear born of misunderstanding. It does not seem that argument should be necessary to fully establish this evident truth.

Worry costs us far more than we realize every day, for it does interfere with every body function; and do not forget that perfect function is perfect health. It is equally true that equable states of the mind, poise, happiness, pleasure, satisfaction with living conditions, tend to stimulate function, to place this on a higher plane.

No, do not be alarmed, the writer is not a Christian Scientist, but a hard-pan Presbyterian of Scottish stock.

He is merely an observer of all the evidences of disease in many types of people, and has perhaps been blessed with more contacts with the ill (if you can call such a blessing) than is given to most men, for he has been treating many thousands of cases from everywhere, not alone in our own country, but from the distant corners of the earth; even South Africa, Japan, China, the Philippines, Russia; everywhere that men think and have heard of a new philosophy that contends that disease is really unimportant, because individually created and fully self-controllable.

It is no more true that fear inhibits body function than that body function deranged through purely physical causes will create fear, for the two are inter-dependent.

Body disarrangement causes fear, and fear depresses and disarranges body function.

We cannot escape such conclusion, if we observe the thing from both angles; and while the metaphysician stresses the mental or fear cause of abnormal physical states, the physician stresses the bodily causes of wrong mental states; both are right and both are equally wrong. It is both conditions, acting on each other, that are to blame for decline in health.

Either alone may be the thing that starts the trouble and

initiates the vicious cycle; and this means that purely physical causes produce fear, and, equally, fear produces physical disharmony.

It is easy enough to say "don't worry," but it is another thing to voluntarily stop worrying; and the worrier is not subject to reason, even admitting that his fears are groundless, yet sticking to them.

This is so notably true of the neurasthenic, the enervated victim of nervous prostration.

Before the break-down that we call by the name of neurasthenia occurs, this vicious cycle has been in operation for some time, and the physician says it has come from digestive or toxic conditions, and the metaphysician says wrong thinking produced the thing, and they never can agree, for each sees as a cause the thing largest in his philosophy.

The writer has observed countless cases of fear that lost all semblance of this handicap when the body was well detoxicated and the diet so arranged as to stop future intoxication.

Many of these were already victims of the so-called nervous breakdown, yet they recovered without exception when the body was well cleared of debris and the formation of this in excess of the eliminative capacity was terminated through correct dietary habit.

It has never yet been his pleasure to see any woman cured of her fear of mice, however, and he is willing to make this one exception. He believes that this fear, as of snakes, is atavistic; born in the race.

But fears of storms, fire, wind, accident, all have been observed to decline and disappear as the body became less toxic.

The case of extreme high blood pressure has a fixed fear of impending calamity, though he has no idea what this calamity is apt to be, and is sure that there is a sword of Damocles hanging over his head continually. He is very toxic, or he could not have high blood pressure; and the treatment necessary to cause decline in blood pressure will also take away his fears.

These blood pressure cases may previously have been men noted for their aggressiveness and energy, but they come into the office and cry like babies over their condition; yet often say they feel fine.

When a man who formerly was optimistic and who accomplished things comes into my office and cries while telling his story, I know he is either a neurasthenic or a high blood pressure case; and the sphygnomanometer applied to the arm soon tells which is the case, for if it is not a high blood pressure then it is a neurasthenia.

Fears! And with a well defined background of purely physical cause in every case, for blood pressure comes always and only from a viscoscity of the blood itself, and this from what we have eaten all of our previous life. The neurasthenia comes from a toxic state also, but not necessarily with high blood viscoscity.

We may not be able to control voluntarily the mental fears, but the body is ours to do with exactly as we mentally decide; and we can keep that from getting into disrepair, and in this way we can prevent fears.

It is hard to think of fear as a physical trait, but having a purely physical cause it is really a physical condition for this reason, and like every disease, it is recognized by its symptoms, or its external signs.

When you find a fearful man or woman you have an individual much less than well. Detoxication and dietary correction will erase the fears just as surely as that removal of fears will improve the body condition; and we see plenty of proof of this.

We have the complete control of fear in our own hands if we but realize it; for a body one hundred per cent well cannot harbor fear.

We are deterred from accomplishing what we should accomplish, by fears and fatigue; both are outgrowths of body intoxication.

Just as surely as you can banish fatigue, just so surely can you banish fears of all kinds by merely creating a body normal in all its parts; and in such a body there is room for neither fatigue nor fear.

This may all seem to you as idle theory, but you can prove to yourself this connection between normal body function and absence of fear very easily.

Start in right away to clean house, either by purging and a fruit fast, or by just the fruit fast, when nothing but fresh fruits is taken for two or three weeks.

Or adopt a wholly alkalin diet for three or four weeks, eating nothing but cooked vegetables, raw vegetable salads, fresh fruits unsweetened, and all the milk or buttermilk desired, and watch the results.

It is not infrequently that quite fixed fears will depart entirely in this rather short time, and tasks that before seemed difficult of accomplishment will soon begin to seem light; while undertakings that one formerly shrank from will be welcomed as something easily overcome.

It will cost nothing to make this test, and it not only will do no harm, but in every way it will do good, as it is merely returning to a more normal state of the body chemistry.

Fear, like disease, is brought about through a saturation of the body with the end-products of digestion and metabolism, the body waste, manufactured in amount greater than can be eliminated daily; and this same accumulation accounts for fatigue, disease, old age, and death.

It has been truthfully said that the only thing to be feared in this world is fear itself; and it is true enough, when we consider that fear is an evidence of body contamination, and when this contamination is cleared away there is no fear.

When fearful you are toxic, and fear this condition as you would the plague itself, for it is the father of all disease.

Visualize any community in which both fear and fatigue are banished, and you will see also a community in which no disease lurks, no hospitals will be there, neither will the insane asylum or the house for defectives flourish. The doctors will be teachers of health, not of disease; and the surgeon will be one who corrects deformities (if such there might be) and repairs wounds from external violence.

Think of the accomplishment possible in such a community, and the pleasures of living possible under such conditions!

This is not Utopian dreaming, but an actual possibility when every individual in any community is so educated in the causes of disease that fear of this is gone, and the means for complete control are well understood and fully in hand.

If the human race were freed from the fear of disease, then surely there would be a better state of affairs.

Let us repeat that with a proper understanding of what disease is and how easily it can be controlled there is not the slightest occasion for fear; and soon there will also be no fear, for without the occasion there will be no resulting effects.

Without fear of disease we can safely plan activities far in the future, for we can have perfect confidence in our ability to keep well all the time.

What would this do to life insurance? First of all it would lower rates, for longevity would increase notably; and it would take away much of the present occasion or need for protection against disease or the abrupt termination of earning capacity, and would accentuate the casualty end of insurance.

Accidents are not always avoidable, as we all realize, so this form of insurance no doubt would be the usual type, and life insurance become of secondary importance, or assume more the role of investment.

With fear of disease removed there would be less financial worries, for our earning capacity rises materially when we are well as we should be, as so many have testified after changing their way of eating.

Mental clearness, alertness, and quick judgment are all assets in business, and their presence or absence may be the determining factors in the size of one's income.

To recite at great length instances of removal of fears of all kinds when dietary habit is changed would no doubt be impressive, but it is scarcely ethical to do so, smacking of the methods of the charlatan.

Rather it is to the point to insist that each make for himself or herself the proof of this easily demonstrated fact; then the proof is self-determined and of vastly more significance than such recital by the writer of this document.

Cases of deeply rooted fears have vanished, and the recipient of this gift from relieved nature is often more impressed with this fact than with the accompanying restoration of normal health.

Many of these have said that they were grateful for the return of abounding health, but were more grateful for the returning sense of freedom from both fatigue and fear; and their mental clearness and alertness was appreciated far more than their physical freedom from disease.

To live in fear is to live under a handicap that is seldom fully realized till relieved; just as we learn to bear physical pain till we almost forget this, and when relieved we then realize the handicap under which we before labored.

When we are fatigued, ill, we fear almost everything that seems to threaten us; we shrink from everything that looks heavy or hard for us and our efficiency suffers, as also our earning power and our enjoyment of living; for we are without zest of life.

When we are functioning up to the normal then life is all zest, all enjoyment; we are ambitious, eager for action, alert, think clearly, make our decisions easily and promptly, and we are then in good position to reap some of the rewards of correct living.

It is pitiful to note the low rate of living of the average man or woman, for so little is accomplished, and this with so little enjoyment, that all seems scarcely worth the effort required.

We realize dimly that our youthful zest is gone, but do not know what to do about it; and all the time we are not as well as nature intended us to be, nor as well as we can be in a few months of correct eating.

Like every other handicap, we scarcely notice this because we have become accustomed to it, even as the north woods guide who can carry a pack of one hundred pounds or more and break trail for his party who are travelling light, seems less fatigued than the rest at night. He has carried packs so long that they do not seem to him heavy; yet the average hunter, untrained in carrying such weight, would find the load of his guide impossible for him to support for more than a very short hike.

We become so accustomed to a sense of fatigue and fear that we scarcely notice this, and realize it only when relieved of both these depressing sensations.

To carry a heavy pack for miles, and then to shift this to the ground makes one feel so light that it seems as though the body is as light as a feather.

One trainer of sprinters made his men wear lead-soled shoes except when running, for this very reason.

These men walked with the heavy gait of old men while off the track, for they were swinging several pounds of lead with each step; but when they were on the track they felt so light that a hard sprint was easy for them.

If we have become accustomed to the usual white man's burden of fatigue and fear, and we suddenly drop this through correct feeding, we feel so light, so competent for anything, that it is small wonder that the recovered man is inclined to accentuate this mental and spiritual lightness above the physical comfort that goes with a clean body.

There is no panacea for fatigue or fear, no medicine that will do more than relieve the sensations; but cure lies in the manner of living.

———•·•———

CHAPTER X.

"Divers Diseases"

WHEN the writer was much younger and less experienced than now, he read of the man in the Bible who suffered from "divers disease," and supposed this referred to disease of deep sea divers.

Diversified disease has always followed the human race, but the diversity in these manifestations has increased and multiplied as medical studies recognized specific forms that seemed to differ sufficiently to warrant separate classification.

Hence description of some supposedly new form of disease was generally tagged with the name of the man who first described it, and thus we have a host of diseases called by the names of their discoverers, as Bright's diseases, Hodgkinson's diseases, Parkinson's diseases, Buerger's disease, Renaud's disease, and many others, each a description of a disease or a symptom-complex. And we have bumptiously called this progress.

The most intimate description of any disease or symptom-complex does nothing to remove this from our literature, but rather perpetuates it; which does nothing for the race.

If such intimate study of disease were to lead directly to means that would eradicate it then indeed would we have the right to crow about our achievements; but no matter how deep our studies, we seem to have an ever-increasing number of conditions recognized as incurable.

The foot gangrene of diabetes we have long recognized as an obliterative end-arteritis, an obliteration of the terminal arteries of the extremities, from retention in the body of certain specific irritants or poisons that are generally peculiar to the state of the diabetic near the finish. Yet, when Dr. Buerger described this as a separate condition, literature immediately attached his name to the description.

118

But this did nothing to cure diabetes or any of the other causes that produce the so-called Buerger's disease.

Since the late war a number of the returned soldiers have suffered this dreadfully painful condition; and either from the free serumization, or the war gasses, this thing has assumed very alarming proportions in the base hospitals, and considered absolutely incurable in every case. Dr. Buerger did nothing but describe the condition as a separate consideration of endarteritis; and while this adds to our knowledge of the condition, yet it does nothing to lessen the suffering of these poor boys, and amputation is still considered the only way out.

It is so with every sort of disease, the intimate study of each seeming to bring us no nearer the therapeutic conquest than before we learned of its intimate pathology. So where is the gain?

It may seem strange to say that all disease is the same thing, no matter what its myriad modes of expression, but it is verily so.

Why do we develop certain diseases, while other seemingly similar mortals develop other forms? If it is true that all disease is one thing, from one source, then why should we not all have the same kinds and degrees of disease? This is a fair question and must have full answer, if you are to be made to understand the unanimity of disease. And this is most important, in order that you may as fully understand the uniformity of treatment for such various conditions as diabetes and tuberculosis, or Bright's disease and asthma, or whooping-cough and mumps.

We inherit from our parents no better bodies than those with which they themselves are equipped; perhaps not so good, for we are apt to inherit all of the deficiencies of both parents.

Our resistance to disease of any sort is predicated on our vitality; our ability to keep close to the normal.

If our parents have already manifested weakness of any

organ, then we will inherit no better resistance of this organ than the parents were able to supply, naturally.

We inherit our facial, physical, and mental characteristics from our parents; also the specific resistance of each organ of the body.

The form of disease we develop is determined by these specific resistances, the least resistant organ acting as our weakest link in the chain of resistance.

So while we might all be equally toxic, the one with weak kidney inheritance will develop Bright's disease, the one with the weak pancreatic inheritance will develop diabetes, the one with the weak skin inheritance will develop skin diseases, the one with the weak pulmonary inheritance will develop bronchial or lung diseases, and the one with weak digestive inheritance will develop digestive disorders.

Hence the divers diseases of the human race, and hence only, if we leave out diversity in living conditions and diversity in dietetic habit, which show a secondary influence on the specificity of disease.

The primary influence, the determining factor usually, is this inherited specific resistance of our individual organs.

If we have some one organ that is not up to par, we have to avoid the causes that tend to lower vitality; and no matter what the organ most weak or most lacking in resistance, we are under necessity of avoiding all the causes of enervation, weakness, or loss of vitality, for when we have dissipated vitality to a point where our weak link is apt to be too severely stressed, we are certain to suffer in this weak link first.

This is our heel of Achilles that represents our chief point of vulnerability, and this must be our index of failure.

The children of tubercular parents do not have to inherit the disease that afflicted their parents, but they do have to conserve vitality in every way if they wish to preserve normal lungs.

The offspring of the diabetic, whether in one or both

parents, do not necessarily die of diabetes, though they are much more apt to do so than the children of those parents who did not suffer from weak pancreatic function.

We can bequeath to our children no better physical equipment than that with which we are ourselves endowed; and this may be stated as a basic truth, one in which all students of heredity are agreed.

It would be as reasonable for a dying parent to bequeath to his children money he did not possess as for him to expect that he could endow his offspring with qualities or quantities of physical perfection that he had not himself enjoyed.

With this fact before us what do we owe our children, in the nature of the physical bequests that we alone are able to furnish?

Any man or woman who seeks to raise a family without a proper physical background of his own is not assisting the development of the physique of the next generation, and is perhaps bequeathing to his children a handicap that will necessitate throughout life the utmost conservation of vitality.

An inheritance of splendid physical resistance is worth infinitely more to any child than a heritage of millions in money.

Not only do parents transmit their own physical qualities to their children, but they also transmit directly a toxic state, which is an immediate handicap during the early years of life.

Yet in spite of this it is still safe to say that any child that is born alive and whole in all its parts, has vitally enough to grow up to adult stature without disease, IF the subsequent feeding habits are correct from the beginning.

That not all children do grow up to adult stature is evidence of the fact that their management subsequent to birth has not been right.

It is this evident fact that accounts for the two hundred thousand deaths before the end of the second year, and the four hundred thousand deaths before the tenth year has passed.

The fact that death rates fall off between the tenth and

fifteenth years does not mean that dietary care has improved, but merely argues a survival of the fittest.

By ten years of age a child has either developed a sufficient or competent resistance, or has failed to do so.

Starting with birth, the intake of nourishment should be such as to supply the body with everything required, and nothing superfluous.

It should always be subject to complete digestion, complete absorption, complete metabolism and complete elimination of resulting debris.

Given such feeding care, and with sufficient sunlight, fresh air, and attention to cleanliness and elimination, any child born alive and whole has every prospect of developing into adulthood in perfect health.

Then why do so many children, born in apparently good health and physical perfection, develop disease and early decline and die?

If we sum up to the final conclusion every possible cause, then those pertaining to the intake of nourishment so far outweigh all the other causes combined that it is almost safe to say that the whole cause of this failure is in wrong feeding habit.

The mother's milk is nature's food for the infant up to two years of age; always supposing that the breast milk is normal, from a normal mother.

This is lamentably untrue, for few mothers are normal, therefore few can furnish normal food for their infants.

Science has devoted great study to the question of the early feeding of infants, and we are still very much in the dark on this most vital subject; but if we stick to the fundamental considerations that pertain to all feeding we shall come close to the correct formula.

Supposing the mother to be deficient in many of the minerals of which the body is made, we are then under necessity of adding in some assimilable form those most likely deficiencies. Orange juice or raw tomato juice offers us the best vehicle for these, both because these juices are tolerated and well digested by the average very young infant, and because either fruit is easily available at almost any season of the year.

Cod liver oil furnishes abundance of the fat-soluble vitamin A, and is a useful addition, not in the usual teaspoonful dose, but five to ten drops once a day, as this small amount does all that the larger amounts would do and without danger of upsetting digestion.

The addition of these two foods to the average breast feeding is safe in every case and does guarantee against the most usual of the deficiencies of early breast feeding.

If the breast milk is not tolerated, or not sufficiently nourishing to the infant, then substitutes must be used. For this there is nothing so good as goat milk, as it more nearly approaches the human standard than does the milk of any other animal; but being much higher in butter fat it requires dilution with sterile water, about fifty-fifty, and this dilution necessitates the addition of small amounts of milk sugar.

If no goat milk is available, then give bovine milk, raw; never the pasteurized kind. This also diluted, as the bovine milk is three times higher in protein or casein than the human standard, and as the bovine infant has a rate of growth three times higher than the human infant.

Use two parts of sterile water to one of the bovine milk; but as both fats and milk sugar have suffered the same dilution as the protein, it becomes necessary to add both cream and milk sugar to the formula.

This humanized bovine milk is thus the easiest substitute for the breast milk. If prepared in this way, and if orange juice is used freely, with the cod liver oil in five to ten drop doses once a day, the parents can feel quite safe about the nutrition of the infant.

The quantity may be too great for competent digestion, so make sure not to go over a pint of milk a day for the first few weeks, which, with the addition of the diluent, would make a quart and a half a day, or much more than the average needs of even a robust baby.

It is perfectly safe to say that most of the deaths of infants are from deficiencies in feeding on the one hand, and the early introduction of starches on the other.

The infant is not equipped for the digestion of concentrated starches till the teeth are all in place.

Teeth are seldom all in place before the end of the second year, so any pediatrist who introduces starchy mushes and gruels before this time is trifling needlessly with the digestion of the baby.

I would say he is trifling dangerously; for constipation, fermentation, acid formation, all arise in the too early introduction of the concentrated starches and sugars, the carbohydrates that are our chief fuels after nature gives us the ptyalin in the salivary secretion to thoroughly split these before they enter the digestive tract.

The ptyalin contained in the saliva of the infant before the advent of full dentition is only sufficient to take care of the milk sugar or the secondary fruit sugars, not sufficient for either cane sugar or starch. It is introducing a needless danger to begin the use of these concentrated and complex forms of carbohydrate before there is full capability for handling them without the dangers that inhere in their use before this period that nature has established.

It is so evident that the milk of the mother is intended for the entire nourishment of the infant for this very reason, that there is not enough ptyalin developed earlier for these concentrated foods, that I see no reason on the part of the pediatrist for ignoring anything so plain.

Deficiencies on the one hand, and impossible tasks in digestion on the other, account for this inexcusable infant mortality of which our medical scientists should be heartily ashamed.

Deficiencies in feeding, together with this too early introduction of concentrated starches and sugars, initiates the divers diseases of later life if it does not terminate life before the later period is reached.

If the little one were born like the "one hoss shay," with no weak places, then the ordinary mistakes in feeding would result in nothing more than digestive disturbances; but with the imperfect physical background of the average infant there will be many weak places in the armour of resistance, and these will tend to give way, the weakest first.

Our heredity determines very largely the form and location of our divers diseases then, and the fact of disease is our own affair.

If we live so as to prevent the accumulation in the system of the acid end-products of digestion and metabolism we will not develop disease of any nature, for there will then be nothing to interfere with the body's processes. If we are born weak in some particular organ we can still live in such a way as to keep within the capacity of this weak link, and so get by year after year, even increasing in general health, till in time we shall be able to forget our imperfect heredity.

The fact of disease itself is that we have accumulated these poisons that interfere with normal function, and the form of the resulting disease is determined by the vitality of each separate organ inherited from our parents.

When we speak of inherited disease we do so with a complete misunderstanding of the thing; for it is impossible to inherit disease, even if we do inherit a predisposition to develop this or that disease through inherited weakness of the organs of resistance.

We so often hear the victim of sick headache excuse herself (it is generally *she* in migraine) by saying that her mother before her had sick headaches, and her grandmother also suffered in this way, therefore the handicap is inherited and must be endured.

This is never true. It is impossible to inherit the makings of headache; for these are always from self-manufactured toxins, and very largely the reabsorption of these from the colon.

You inherit the colon from the mother, but the manner of caring for the colon is up to you; also the liver is inherited, but the decay of food residues in the colon that has caused the liver to be less than an efficient organ, is self-created always.

Certain diseases are supposed to "run in families." This is partially accounted for by inheritance of organs less than efficient, but similar family habit of eating is also a large factor.

It is not only possible to live with a poor inheritance so as to achieve perfect health and long life, but it is a certain fact that we can do this in every case if we eat right and do not neglect the other natural adjuvants to health, as sun, air, water, exercise, sleep.

Not only is it certain that this can be accomplished, but there are numerous instances of individuals who have started with the worst possible heredity and yet who have succeeded in developing a wonderful physique and superb health that continued to a good old age.

Heredity is the water that has passed under the bridge. We cannot concern ourselves with this, for no matter what we might do we are powerless to change our heredity.

The comforting fact, however, is that no matter how poor this heritage of resistance may be, we still can live in perfect health and to a ripe old age by never conflicting the immutable laws of our being in the matter of eating and general living.

Not only can we guarantee ourselves this but we can have far more enjoyment in life than we have ever thought possible.

Medical so-called science treats these various manifestations of disease, and seems to believe that this is all that can be done about it; in fact it resents any other view; and medicine is always pictured as warring against disease, which means these manifestations of disease.

There is no treatment under the sun that can add one atom of resistance to any organ, for resistance is determined by our heredity plus our manner of living; and just as surely as medicine cannot make the hair grow, or restore a missing part, or replace a fingernail, just so surely can medicine do nothing constructive for any disease.

Medicine may change the symptoms, relieve pain, cause the bowels to move with the usual whip of laxatives; it may so occupy our imagination as to delude us into thinking that our condition is better after the exhibition of a remedy than before; but in any way to change the condition of the body for the better is not in the function of therapeutics. Nature creates, maintains and regulates the organs; and nature alone can mend them when broken, though medicine may make this repair process less disagreeable.

Can you not see that it is very largely a waste of precious time to go so deeply into the study of manifestations of disease? No possible amount of study can change the thing for the better, for nature alone can do this.

It is enough to know that the body has departed from the normal condition, and it is significant to note the extent of this departure; but the main thing is to know the way back; and whether we ignore the form of manifestation, or whether we concentrate on this all of our attention, really makes no difference in the final result. All that counts is removal of the deterrents to natural recovery, which can be done whether we have a minute picture of the present pathology or whether we fail to see this at all.

This brings us back to the statement made before, that after all, disease is one thing, merely a departure from the normal through certain well known paths; and when these are known, so also will the way back to health be known; for successful treatment surely consists in a complete reversal of those causes that produced the departure from health.

So however diverse our diseases, let us not lose sight of the fact that there is back of all of them one underlying cause that must be removed before we can consider ourselves on the way back to health; and that the specific form of this departure from health matters little, if we but recognize the facts of departure and the way by which we departed; and this all precedent to the knowledge of the way we are compelled to take if we would reverse the causes of disease and eventually arrive at the desired termination, health.

We hope to show you the way of departure and the way back; the means by which we have become less than well, and the simplicity of the road that leads us back to nothing less than freedom from all disease.

CHAPTER XI.

The Practice of Medicine

WE are all familiar with what is meant by the phrase, "The Practice of Medicine;" and it must be that the ancients had in mind that the application of medicines to human ills is always in the nature of practice.

If practice always made perfect then we could be resigned to the use of this word till the physician reached perfection in his efforts to relieve the ills of suffering humanity.

But, however extensive or long continued the practice, it does not seem to result in anything better than the beginnings, except as it does in some cases so impress the practitioner with the uselessness of drug administration as to make him afraid to administer any remedy that might in any manner influence the body for the worse instead of for the better. In this case practice has made better, if not perfect.

Some physicians of all time have recognized the uselessness of the administration of drugs, and have warned against the indiscriminate use of those drugs or chemicals that might influence the body deleteriously; but the average physician takes his materia medica very seriously, and in large doses, not for his own use, but for his patients'.

Below we will quote at length from an address delivered by Dr. Robert Hutchinson, F.R.C.P., before the British Academy of Medicine, and published in the British Medical Journal, under date of May 30th, 1925. What he said there and then can be said just as truthfully here and now.

It was in regard to the presence of fads in medical practice, and follows:

"The perfectly natural desire on the part of the doctor to 'prove all things' is also responsible for keeping fashions going for a time. He is not sure that 'there may not be something in it.' This attitude of mind is perfectly laudable; but other motives by no means laudable are sometimes at work also, for truth compels one to admit that there are a few members of our profession who exploit fashions and play up to the public demands for them because it pays so to do. This unsavory aspect of our subject I do not propose to dwell on, but I think few will deny that it exists.

It is bad enough in all conscience, that the saying 'doctors differ' should have become a proverb. But it is worse still that we should exhibit such a collective variability in our views and practice from year to year; that we should at one time attribute most human ills to uric acid, at another to auto-intoxication, to oral sepsis, to disturbance of the endocrine balance, or to avitaminosis; that our pathological beliefs should be dominated now by toxins, now by reflex action, or by vicious cycles; that today we should seek to cure all manner of disease by excising the ovaries; tomorrow, by removal of the appendix or the teeth; one year by injection of sea-water, another by the administration of sour milk, or by the application of violet rays; that we should pin our faith for collective salvation sometimes to team work, and at other times to early diagnosis or preventive medicine; in short, that we should be as much at the mercy of 'stunts' as the yellow press, as much the slaves of catchwords as politicians, and as intellectually unstable as the popular electorate.

It is commonly said that education is a great safeguard against quackery and faddery. I profoundly disbelieve it. So far as I can see, the higher one goes in the social scale the more does fashion in health matters prevail, and the so-called intelligentsia are the most gullible of all, and it would almost seem, indeed, as if everyone has a certain stock of credulity, and the more sceptical

THE PRACTICE OF MEDICINE

he is in everything else the more credulous he is in matters medical. It may be replied that this is the wrong kind of education, and what is needed is more teaching of science. Again I disbelieve. If this were so the saying of Matthews Duncan would not be true — as I, for one, believe it to be — that 'there are more quacks inside the profession than outside of it'."

This is from the pen of a man who knows medicine and sees its limitations too plainly for the comfort of his medical brethren. Yet it was this same man who at Toronto recently set at rest once and forever, as he evidently supposed, the question of incompatibilities in certain foods, by quoting the old saying that nature never makes mistakes, and as nature combines in one food both protein and starch, therefore it cannot be wrong to eat these dissimilar food materials in combination.

Perhaps if he tried separating these incompatibles for a time he would not inquire so diligently for the reasons for medical faddery and disagreement, or why stunts and fashions spring up in the practice of medicine.

Like every other critic of medicine he can point the imperfections but cannot point the remedy; an iconoclast but never a constructionist.

It is well denominated the "practice of medicine;" and till something is known and taught of the fundamental underlying causes of all disease there still will be fads and fashions, for practice does not yet include the correction of predisposing causes of disease.

It is this misunderstanding of disease and its origin that has led to the creation of specialties, each treating but one manifestation of disease, and each superfluous if the universal cause is removed.

An old and very wise Philadelphia physician was called as a witness in a law suit, and placed on the stand as an expert.

The opposing counsel was inclined to belittle his qualifications as a witness in this particular case, as the doctor said he did not specialize in any one condition of disease, being an internist, one who treats all disease, not one particular phase of disease.

The attorney asked him what the difference was between a specialist and general practitioner; and the doctor replied that it took seventeen kinds of doctors to fill the specialties and it took them all to make one general practioner; which was not far from the truth.

What else can be expected when men are thoroughly trained in all the possible aberrations in function of but one organ? To such a man the body is all this one organ, and he is sure it is abnormal if not found in the classical state prescribed by authorities in this specialty.

As the various medical specialties have multiplied even so have diseases multiplied; for thorough training will so exaggerate the possible deviations from the normal that it is not to be expected that one can go to the throat specialist and be told that his throat is normal, neither can he go to the oculist and expect to leave there without glasses.

The heart is such a misunderstood organ that it is easy for the specialist in heart disease to find some slight abnormality in almost every heart presented for treatment. If you have never been told that you have something wrong with your heart it must be because you have not had occasion to consult the heart specialist, or else he was not in when you called.

The heart is merely a part of the body, and it does reflect the troubles that afflict the whole man, perhaps even more directly than do most of his organs, for it is one organ that has little time for rest.

With most heart specialists heart disease and digitalis are almost synonymous terms, for the two are connected so intimately in his thought that it is hard to dissociate them

Yet digitalis has but one use in heart conditions and this

[132]

is in acute dilations, where it does stimulate the heart to more efficient contraction, but it does nothing to remove the causes of the dilation. If these causes are mechanical, they still persist, for the digitalis cannot restore a leaking valve. If they are nutritional, as they so frequently are, still digitalis does nothing to change the body chemistry to the normal, and again it is merely a whip to stimulate function for a time, leaving the chemistry as chaotic as before.

Heart disease treated as any other disease, by correction of the chemistry of the whole man, disappears as does every other manifestation of body failure, with the exception of the valvular lesions, which are not usually changed by correction of the nutrition. Yet even these do disappear, if the dilation is the result of weakening of the heart muscle, instead of from a previous crippling of the valvular mechanism.

If the extra work entailed as a result of a former destruction of a valve through inflammation has caused the dilation, then it is not to be supposed that proper feeding habits will correct this; but if wrong nutrition of the body has weakened the heart to the point of dilation of its chambers, then indeed can this whole condition be corrected by restoring chemical balance, as has been witnessed times without number.

This is not the practice of medicine, but a recognition of the underlying causes and their removal, thus giving nature opportunity to restore the heart muscle as nature alone is able to restore.

The ideal practice of medicine is observance of all the departures from the normal, and removal of all the obstacles to a return to the state of body intended by nature. This is a let-alone practice, largely, for there is little that can be done but wait, after the evident obstacles to recovery are removed.

Not infrequently the most heroic thing that can be done is to wait, however hard this seems to be. It is perfectly natural for the friends, perhaps also the patient, to feel that "something ought to be done" to antagonize the disease, to eradicate it completely, little realizing that every disease is merely the price we are paying for our failure to live according to the divine plan of nature herself, and that we cannot get back to the normal at once, but must let nature herself work out the plan of return in her own way.

We offend nature all of our lives, and we pay, not occasionally, but always and infallibly, whether we realize this or not.

To recover from disease of any kind is to stop all the infractions of natural law, nothing more or less; and to attempt to recover from disease without cessation of the infractions that have caused the thing is as futile as bailing a leaky boat without first stopping the leak.

Without this continual warfare against disease the physician can be of vastly more use to his patient if he discovers in what ways the body has offended against nature, how far it has gone toward the final reckoning of account, how much damage has been done, and just what must occur before the body can again hope to function normally.

This is the legitimate practice of medicine, and not merely the analysis of the body condition at the time and the ineffectual application of so-called remedies for the various symptoms, whether this be from the standpoint of the internist or the surgeon.

If we realize that when we offend we pay, somewhere, sometime, we will be the more careful not to offend.

The application of man-made laws does not carry infallible punishment for every infraction, even though this is prescribed; for it is necessary first to catch the offender, then to build up a chain of evidence that will warrant conviction, before punishment is meted out.

Nature's laws are not so, for they do not have to catch the offender, and the evidence is self-contained and complete from the beginning.

The punishment always fits the crime in nature's administration, and injustice is never present here.

[134]

There is never vicarious administration of punishment, but each is punished infalliby for the sins against his or her own body. Neither can there be vicarious relief from punishment, each infraction of law being punished on the body of the infractor.

When we apply to the physician for treatment we are seeking vicarious relief from our past sins against the body; and if we remember that there is no such thing it will help us to see the folly of spending money and wasting time to do something that only we can do in the end.

Accidents, malformations of the body, are things against which we have no protection except the chance of fate; for we cannot control our heredity, neither can we always escape external violence. To the surgeon who attends to both of these accidents we owe all the honor and gratitude that belong to the surgical body generally, for it is these men who are doing constructive work.

To the curiosity of the internal surgeon, the one who opens the hermetically sealed cavities of the body under the pretext of doing something that will benefit us in some way, we owe nothing; but against him we can charge much of the misery of post-operative conditions; and the world is well-filled today with surgical wrecks.

If those occasions in which surgical intervention is indicated in internal conditions could be well defined, we would be shocked to find that these are but a pitiful fraction of one per cent of the whole. If we knew that surgery is responsible for more deaths today than any one disease, more than the losses of the late war, even, we would not be so inclined to fall for the blandishments of the urbane surgeon who tells us that we need an internal operation, and that without this we can carry on but a short and hazardous time.

Again fear is the weapon used, and only because the natural fear of internal operations is overcome by the greater fear of dire calamity and early death predicted by the surgeon, who, we are taught to suppose, makes no mistakes.

Appendicitis is supposed to be an essentially surgical condition, and to hint that there is another possible aspect is to incur the lasting disrespect and wrath of any surgeon. Yet in the practice of the writer, (himself formerly sold to the surgical idea in appendicitis), during the past twenty-six years there has not been one death from any form of this very common accident.

No surgery was invoked in any case, even in the ruptured cases, numbering nineteen. Nothing was done except to empty the colon as completely as possible and withhold everything from the digestive tract, even water, till the resulting abscess had matured and emptied again into its natural point of least resistance—the colon itself.

When rupture of the appendix occurs there is at once a formation of adhesive bands about the area, sequestering this completely; and it is unthinkable that nature can do this instantaneous job and then fail to maintain this barrier.

The surgeon opens the abdomen, breaks up this restraining wall of adhesions, and in doing so opens fresh lymph channels to further infection; and fifty per cent of his ruptured cases die, as he expects, but his ready alibi is always that the case was operated on too late.

The very latest operation for ruptured appendix is much too early, for surgical interference at any stage introduces many dangers not in the simple process of emptying the colon and waiting till nature has evacuated the abscess into this sewer.

Nineteen cases of ruptured appendix is not a large number, to be sure, but till one death occurs from this simple and sane mode of treatment I am sure it is possible to excuse the attitude taken by the writer, that waiting is far safer than to rush in where angels should fear to tread.

In all, over four hundred cases of every type and degree

of appendicitis have gone through this simple process of emptying of the colon and correcting the diet, without one failure, or one case that has had to go through operative treatment.

Appendicitis comes from the character of the colon contents, and surgical removal of the damaged organ, appendix, does not alter the cause.

The practice of medicine and surgery is the treatment of disease after it has become recognizable as disease, and it is in the nature of a locking of the stable door after the horse has been stolen, never in any sense a constructive proceeding, and far too often destructive.

This is especially true if in the drug treatment of disease some so-called remedy is used that remains in the body, as minerals of all kinds are quite apt to do.

This is destructive to function if anything has been introduced that in any way hampers the body's own methods of maintaining its own work level. Even if this mineral is nothing more than the familiar baking soda, there is interference with the body's processes; or if it is the well known magnesia, so advertised as an ideal antacid, still this is also in mineral form, and sure to remain long in the body.

The body does not well tolerate foreign substances of any kind, and the fact that the normal body contains both soda and magnesium does not alter the case, for these are in colloidal form, and in no other form can the body handle chemicals.

Nature does not produce any minerals in food form, except those in the form of colloids, whether in fruit, vegetable, nut or grain.

The surgical treatment of disease is destructive always, except in the correction of deformities and the repair of wounds.

To open the abdominal cavity is to break into a hermetically sealed pocket of the body, and no surgeon is smart enough to in any way improve on nature's arrangements there, even though he can drain abscesses, remove inflamed organs, break

[137]

up adhesions, anchor ptosic viscera to the wall, none of which can compare with nature's own arrangements for repair, IF we cease to cause the conditions which surgery is seeking to correct.

It is not enough that the patient survives the ordeal of surgery, for it takes more than this to kill many individuals; and survival is no guarantee that the operation was justifiable, neither that it was a success; though any operation is supposed to be successful if the surgeon can complete it before death.

Many a case has died within a day or two following operation as a direct result of the surgical procedure, or indirectly through infection of the peritoneum; yet this death is never charged to the operation, but is considered one of those distressing contingencies for which there was no preventive.

The public has become so used to the almost daily reports of death following operation that this is not news; and all seem to feel that at least surgery gave the sufferer a chance, when, if the truth were known, it would be found that the death should have been charged to the operation.

If every surgeon were compelled to post a sizable bond before opening any of the body cavities, a bond that would guarantee to leave conditions as good after the operation as before, no better, it would soon cut down reckless surgery to very modest proportions, and the front page would be without so much morgue news.

If operation is undertaken for conditions that can be better controlled through other means, it is a serious thing indeed to subject the patient to the immediate danger of internal operation, and to the almost certainty of worse conditions after than before this vandalism.

It is a question of indemnity, but try to get it, and you will find that no matter how seriously the operation threatened the life or usefulness of the patient, so long as he consented to it, and providing that the surgeon is properly registered and can show the required credentials, he is immune to prosecution anywhere in our country; or if prosecuted he can present a host of reputable professional witnesses who will glibly swear that the operation was necessary and that surgery alone was the answer; also that the operator was well qualified and performed the operation in approved manner and form; so where would you be if you were seeking indemnity? May the Lord speed the day of less internal surgery.

CHAPTER XII.

The Proof of the Pudding

THE writer is no magician or worker of miracles, neither does he claim the slightest credit for recovery in any case he accepts for treatment. He realizes far more keenly than do most, that recovery is a function of the body alone, and that nature, as represented by the body, has her own ways for repairing this useful automaton when out of order. So all any human being can do is to successfully interpret nature and give her what assistance is possible in the way of removal of the visible handicaps to her work.

He has the Scotch habit of insisting that two and two should always make four, and if otherwise, then he is being "gypped."

It took fifteen years of patient and persistent application of the principles here laid out to remove finally and definitely from his mind all specificity of disease, and to enable him to regard all diseases as one thing, subject to the same rules and requiring the same form of treatment.

To him now a toothache is merely an evidence of wrong chemical conditions of the body, conditions that he believes he can suggest as universal in all departures from health.

Progressive pernicious anaemia, asthma, Bright's disease, diabetes, rheumatism, arthritis, neuritis, gastric or duodenal ulcer, every form of digestive disturbance, eczema, psoriasis, pityriasis, goitres of all types, tumors, tuberculosis, — any and all of these varied forms of so-called disease fall under one head,—chemical imbalance of the body; and all are subject to restoration to the normal through correction of the body chemistry and thorough drainage.

This is a radical simplification of the consideration of disease, and takes it out of the realm of mystery.

The very fact that all these varied conditions recover to a

high normal is surely proof enough of the correctness of the theory, and it matters nothing that high authority says these things are wholly unmanageable by any known form of treatment.

Such statement merely proves that the so-called authority does not know the cause of these conditions, therefore is not a good guide for anyone seeking relief.

When the best that medical science can do for any of the conditions mentioned above is to temporize, treat symptoms, and recognize them all as incurable, surely there must be something wrong with their ideas of the origin of any of them and how to correct them.

To regard disease as merely a departure from normal health, no matter what form this departure takes, simplifies its consideration so greatly that it does not require medical training to appreciate it fully, nor anything resembling talent to find means for its relief, as the understanding of the thing carries automatically with it the knowledge of how to return to health.

It was said earlier that all we can do for disease is to stop creating this background of acid end-products of digestion and metabolism; and this is true; for if disease comes always and only from this acid collection, then it must be evident to anyone that the cure lies in the discontinuance of this accumulation.

Septic troubles of all kinds yield to simple dextoxication and dietary correction wholly without sera or drugs or anything else.

In deep types of blood poisoning the use of three heaping tablespoonfuls of Epsom or Glauber salts, or a half pint of concentrated Pluto water on an empty stomach, repeated if necessary for three or more days, and with diet of nothing but water or surely nothing more than orange juice or other unsweetened juice, has not to this very date failed to restore the body to a near enough normal so that the temperature has subsided, and appetite has returned, usually within two or three days, even after antistreptococcic serum had been used and

[141]

many forms of medication, without regulation of the diet or detoxication by purging.

Temperature ranging up to 105 F., with chills, delirium, collapse, the count of the white cells enormous, have after two to three days shown normal temperature, have rapidly come back to normal, and showed a very high degree of health afterward, with no sequelae remaining to tell of the stresses of the past two weeks.

Pneumonia, erysipelas, typhoid fever, influenza, acute arthritis, colitis, hay fever, all subside when the body is fairly detoxicated and the diet so corrected as to stop this excessive formation of the acid end-products, simply because each is expressing the end-point of tolerance for toxins, and each is the means by which the body seeks to unload this unwanted mass.

The acute fevers of little children pass in one night as a rule, leaving the little one wanting food the very next day. No matter how small the child, this crisis means always the same thing, which is that the little body has accumulated toxins to the point of tolerance and is now trying to unload by means of a fever, or heightened oxidation process, during which much of this waste is burned and thrown out.

Little children can scarcely be made to take the nauseating dose of salts or Pluto water, so the tasteless castor oil is better here, using double the prescribed dose in every case.

The object of the purge is not the movement of the bowels, though this is accomplished also, but it is intended to remove from the body much of its acid-laden fluids, the serum from the blood, the lymph from the tissues.

In the adult the use of a half pint of concentrated Pluto water will usually result in the ejection from the bowel of three or four quarts of fluid; and the thirst resulting from this dehydration will make the free use of fruit juices very gratifying. Thus an alkalin or base-forming source of supply is opened up for the body to replenish its deficient stores; and the condition of the body immediately is one of lowered acidity, or rather a heightened alkalinity.

This is neutralizing much of the mass of acid end-products, hence the feeling of relief that usually follows this rather drastic purging; and the more toxic the condition the greater the feeling of relief.

Many cases of nephritis, with broken heart compensation, unable to walk about through weakness, unable to lie down because of the shortness of breath, will purge for three days and then lie down flat to sleep and even take walks with enjoyment; all without any food whatever.

Always before coming under treatment an effort had been made to "keep up the strength" with foods of all sorts; yet in spite of this free feeding they were extremely weak, while after this spasm of intensive detoxication they were stronger at once, without food.

This would seem to indicate that the weakness formerly was from the intoxication, and the relief of this by the drastic purge allowed of better function at once, accounting for the seeming increase in strength. Surely there seems to be no other way to look at it.

Nephritis, or Bright's disease as it is usually called, is one of the very deep types of intoxication, and what is accomplished there is duplicated by the before-mentioned blood infections, as streptococcic infection, or so-called blood poisoning, where the immediate relief from the purge and fast or near-fast, is rather impressive, especially to one who is familiar with the usual course of these unmanageable conditions.

True anginas, whether from degenerative changes in the heart muscle or from embolism of the coronary artery, will generally lose all pain on exertion after three days of active purging and fruit juice diet, go on to complete relief, even returning to active exercise, golf, even tennis, and with no remaining evidence of heart incompetency.

Every case of arthritis short of actual anchylosis, or fixation of joints, will respond to treatment. Complete recovery is the rule, not the exception, the result limited only by the degree of fixation of the joints.

Many a case of gastric or duodenal ulcer responds at once, the very first day of fruit juices bringing grateful relief; but in those cases of bleeding ulcer it is not wise to use the drastic purge to start the detoxication period, for fear of exciting haemorrhage.

It is enough to empty the colon daily by means of the simple enema and confine the food wholly to the fruit juices till all pain has completely subsided, then begin feeding with the wholly alkalin foods, as cooked vegetables, raw vegetable salads, fresh fruits, and a moderate amount of milk or buttermilk, the latter preferred.

To date no case of gastric or duodenal ulcer has failed to entirely recover, though some go through several recurrences, usually each lighter and shorter than preceding attacks; but the thing is cyclic in character, and tends to return at intervals of six months to one year, a few cases having cycles of two years, when the attack comes on, is severe for a time, then gradually subsides, no one knows why; but it is thinkable that the pain of digestion so limits the intake of food that in time there is relief from the irritation that produces the trouble. If it were not for the fact that the victim when relieved of pain returns to his former incompatible habits of eating he would not suffer recurrences; but when the history is long, and there have been many cycles, the cause is so deeply rooted that even correct eating may not be sufficient to guarantee freedom from recurrences till the body's chemistry is well changed. However, each case recovers ultimately, proving that a hyper-acid state of the body was the cause, for only alkalinization of the body was required for cure.

The late Dr. Sippy, of Chicago, who specialized in the treatment of gastric and duodenal ulcer for many years, made the statement on the floor of the Erie County Medical Society not long before his death, that every case of gastric or duodenal ulcer was orginally a hyperchlorhydria, meaning that a too free production of hydrochloric acid in the gastric juice was the active irritant in every case.

The writer's experience fully bears out this statement of Dr. Sippy; but the so-called Sippy diet, or bland diet, while it does give relief, never ultimately cures, for there is always a tendency to recurrence of the cycles till the whole body chemistry is changed to a more alkalin state, a thing Dr. Sippy did not believe. Hence his cases returned to him again and again with recurrences, while if the diet had been sufficiently alkalin throughout, very few cases would have ever suffered relapse, and in time all cases would have recovered permanently.

The word "permanently" is used advisedly, though it carries with it the understanding that a repetition of the former wrong habits of eating would insure a return of the ulcer.

One hundred and nine cases of progressive pernicious or primary anaemia passed through the same simple form of detoxication and dietary correction, and all but eight recovered; the eight simply being too far gone to permit of time for the necessary changes.

In every recovery the result was permanent except in those who returned to careless habit of diet and neglected to thoroughly empty the colon every day.

Of course a repetition of the original causes would naturally tend to produce the same result, as the original attack showed the weak link in the chain of resistance, and a similar toxic condition would be quite likely to express through this same weak point.

Primary or progressive pernicious anaemia is a failure of the blood-making organs, as against a secondary anaemia, which is due to destruction of the red cells from some internal or external toxic material; and the secondary type disappears when this source of destruction is found and corrected.

The primary type has long been considered a mystery, and

no one attempted to tell the origin of the influence that depressed the function of the blood-making organs.

The chronic asthmatic, the spasmodic type, is probably the most grateful and the most greatly surprised of all chronic sufferers, for usually he has been everywhere, has tried everything, has consulted the best specialists, and has been told everywhere that nothing can be done for him except to send him to a higher and dryer climate, and usually this also is found to give but little and temporary relief.

The very first week, in the majority of cases, shows marked relief from spasm; and in the case of young children even a week is more than is necessary to show this, for many of them never again have the slightest sign of asthma after even less than a week following three days of drastic purging and alkalin diet.

The relief seems to the asthmatic almost unbelievable, but it is not well to promise such speedy relief in the beginning, for this sufferer has gone through too much to believe easily that his trouble of years past has been all this time such a simple thing; then, too, his may be one case that requires a longer time, as some rare cases do.

So the asthmatic is told that his case is curable if he will follow faithfully the directions given; and if he is one of the lucky ones and loses his whole trouble in the first few weeks of treatment he will be the happiest man in the world.

Spasmodic or catarrhal asthma is nothing but a toxic state expressed through bronchial tubes that are not any too large at best. It does not require much swelling of these little capillary tubes to seriously interfere with their function of carrying air into the lungs and carbonic acid gas out, and so the victim smothers from this difficulty.

As the hyper-acid state subsides so does the catarrhal swelling everywhere, while a little subsidence in the tiny bronchial tubes does make a great deal of difference in the breathing of anyone.

It was not long ago that we began to recognize colitis as the frequent occurrence that it really is; and now we understand that every case of constipation is a colitis of degree, whether mucus is thrown off or not. Colitis is now regarded as so common that in almost every case presented for treatment there will be found evidence of catarrh of the colon in some degree, just as we expect that few people will be able to say that they have the natural three bowel movements daily.

If mucus is not observed in the stools it soon will be after the beginning of daily enemata and the correction of the diet to a more alkalin standard. This first appearance usually leads the patient to think that the enema or the diet is doing harm; but the opposite is the case. The body is only beginning to unload this waste material, and the more mucus the better the indication, for this is accentuated elimination, and should go on till no more mucus is left to show in the stools.

Colitis comes from the character of the contents of this neglected organ; a toxic mass, putrefying, fermenting, is retained too long, and unless the colon is emptied daily there will continue to be absorption from this sewer, and recovery will be delayed till it is borne in on the patient's mind that it is better to get this material out than to let it remain to further putrefy and ferment.

There is not the slightest chance of permanently injuring the function of this organ by our doing its work vicariously for a time, because its function depends on internal cleanliness as much as on anything else, though ultimate recovery of normal bowel tone is a matter of general revitalization of the whole body, and till this has had time to occur it will be necessary to continue to aid this burdened organ in this way.

Every case of colitis recovers if the diet is correct and if the colon contents are daily flushed out by the simple enema till such time as returning general vitality restores the tone of every organ and part of the body, a period that varies from a few weeks to a few months in most cases; but in constipation of deep type and long history it may require two, three, or more years to regain a competent activity of the colon.

Next to constipation the common cold is perhaps the thing most prescribed for and least understood.

The P. H. S. undertook an intensive study of colds some time ago, I believe at the suggestion of the president. That this will accomplish anything is too much to expect, for there is little or nothing known about the real cause of this very common condition.

The cold will never be properly understood till we realize that each attack is merely the body's end-point of tolerance for the acids of digestion and metabolism, and when we have ceased to create these toxic materials we will cease to manifest the common cold.

When patients have kept the colon well up to the minute and have so corrected their dietary habit as to stop this excessive formation of adventitious acids, no more colds will be manifested, and in a few years no possible exposure can again produce this manifestation that we call a cold. Were this not true then everything before said would fall flat; for here is a very good way to prove the whole thing; and one would not dare to make any such statement as that colds will become impossible when the body has raised its alkalinity to anywhere near the normal, unless able to prove it.

Eat all foods compatibly, bring the colon up to date, and you will furnish yourself with all the proof necessary that it becomes impossible for you to "catch cold."

Colds are not caught; they are accumulated with the feet under the dinner table, and in no other way.

If you will stop creating the usual acid excesses and keep the colon up to date, you will find plenty of other reasons to point to the general fact that disease of every sort comes from accumulation of these acid end-products of digestion and metabolism. you will be abundantly impressed with the proof of all of the foregoing, and will begin to realize that after all old mother nature is your very best friend.

You have not listened to her in the past or you would have long ago discovered this. Start right in today to listen hard to all her suggestions, and you will come to have the most profound respect for her.

It has often been said that nature is a very good nurse, but a poor physician; and this is true enough, if by physician you mean one who treats disease; for she does not treat disease, and neither should we.

We should ignore disease and concentrate on building health; which means that we should not fail to observe all the natural indications of the body in health or its opposite, and satisfy ourselves with keeping the laws of our own nutrition, and we will need only a nurse, and nature is after all the very best.

Sir William Osler once said that anything that can not be cured by nature must forever remain uncured; which would seem to indicate that he considered the old lady not only the best of nurses, but not so bad as a physician also.

It is safe to say that of all the thousands of cases that have been presented here for the past twenty-six years, by far the largest number were those who had gone through almost every form of so-called treatment at the hands of many physicians, but who, like the poor woman in the Bible had spent all their substance, and grew nothing better, but rather grew worse. With few exceptions these have regained their lost health in part or in whole, and at the same time have learned the blessed lesson that as we eat so are we; and they have been able since to conform sufficiently to the body's laws so as to guarantee their health for the future.

It is good to recover from supposedly unmanageable disease, but it is better, in a far larger way, to know why one has been less than well, and just how to conserve the health and vitality for the future.

[149]

This I consider constructive therapeutics—nothing else is; and till official medicine takes similar ground they should not complain if the public is losing confidence in their treatment of disease, and is turning to Osteopaths and Chiropractors, or even to Christian Science—the last abjuring all forms of treatment.

CHAPTER XIII.

Correct Eating Habits

TO visualize absolutely correct eating habits we will probably have to return to a study of original man in normal environment, surrounded by nothing but natural foods, and under no necessity to conform to habits of his neighbors that may be far from normal.

Keeping up with the Joneses has caused many a break-down in those who are not of independent mind, or who cannot think independently or reason correctly.

Man in his original habitat, and before habits of eating had so changed his chemistry that no normal desire was prevalent, no doubt ate when hungry and of the things which were at hand, selecting from these the foods that particularly appealed to his sense of taste at the time. He no doubt ate all he desired at the time, but did not again seek food till hunger suggested a search.

It would be extremely easy under such primitive conditions to keep the body in normal health; but today our conditions are very far from the primitive; and convention has so prescribed our lives that we seldom stop to think much about ourselves, or to study ourselves apart from the mob, or to see what it is that we particularly need at the time.

Conventional meal time, conventional foods and conventional menus dominate our choice, so that there is little left for individual preference.

When we see one menu of almost any first class hotel we see them all; for each contains almost everything usually eaten, and also much that is seldom called for.

Even the order of courses is almost identical in all; and to really depart from this is to excite criticism, or to inspire the idea that we may not be up to date in customary eating.

Food for the active and the sedentary may contain the same

things, but in vastly different proportions, the active requiring much of the fuel foods, as starches, sugars, fats, while the sedentary one needs little of these.

Protein needs are identical in both classes, as protein is for but one purpose, and that is the replacement of our own tissues; and as these die and need replacement at an even rate, whether we are active or sedentary, we all need protein in proportion to our size, not our activity.

So the diet of the active may contain, or should contain, a much larger proportion of the breads, cereals, starches, sugars, fats, than that of his less active neighbor.

To eat because it is dinner time, or because we have heard the noon whistles, is to fall a victim to habit; and if it is wrong to be a clock-watcher at work, it is even worse to eat in the same way.

Our needs from day to day are not uniform, even though our activities compare closely one day with another. The body stores a part of foods eaten, and may have enough stored up to last for a day or two without replacement; so some days we have little desire for food, and other days we seem to need a great deal.

We should respect this variation in desire, and conform our habit to this, even as the animals always do, or as the primitive man would surely do.

This habit of waiting for hunger before taking any nourishment need not interfere with the regular meal hours in the least; for when we are not hungry we can still go to the table for sociability's sake, but we do not need to eat the bill, only so much as we feel actually hungry for.

Many have said that they have never known normal hunger for food, but always ate because it was meal time, or because of the insistence of the hostess or the cook.

Such have never known really good health unless they have eaten very moderately of the right foods; and one eating so is seldom able to make complaint against feeble appetite.

As the body through its various activities uses up its stores of fuels, it expresses the need for fresh fuels through hunger, not conventional appetite; for appetite is a creation of habit, and comes at the usual hours for taking nourishment, while hunger is a real expression of need for food.

Appetite is accompanied by a disagreeable sensation of "goneness" or sinking in the stomach, and is the irritation of acid debris left from the last meal. If you wish to prove this, take a teaspoonful of baking soda or a tablespoonful of milk of magnesia and you will note the disappearance of this sinking sensation; proving that it did not express a need for food, but a discomfort from acid debris.

Eating relieves this sensation, of course, because it dilutes this debris; but each indulgence merely creates a higher degree of acid and requires earlier and more complete dilution of the debris. In this way we build up a fearfully acid state of the stomach and the entire body by creating such amounts of acid end-products.

Hunger is to tell us when we need food, as thirst is to tell us when we need fluids. Unless we have hunger we need no food at the time; and unless we are thirsty we need no drink, else nature is all out of tune; and the man who tells you that you need to take three quarts of water every day whether you desire this or not is after all right, and nature is the blind guide that he thinks her.

If we wish to cultivate normal eating habits we will stay away entirely from all unnatural foods, those unfit to eat till changed from their original form; for only so can we expect to cultivate again a normal sense that will tell us when we are hungry and what we should eat.

All animals in their normal state have this instinct; but man has so civilized himself that he no longer can be guided by this natural instinct that guides the animal, but must eat as custom dictates, hoping this is right, but really not having

[153]

ability to think fundamentally or reason correctly, so compelled to follow the crowd.

Wait till distinctly hungry before taking nourishment of any kind, and then take the thing you most desire, IF this is natural food, not something refined or manufactured.

If you are satisfied with this one article, all the better; but if you still desire something else, make sure that it conforms to the same chemical requirements as the original food taken; and if a third is craved this too must conform to chemical laws of the other two, else chaos in digestion will result, with much fermentation and acid formation.

The writer has in mind several people who travel extensively, who eat in every foreign country where the tourist seeks relief from the monotony of civilized life, yet who are able to conform to nearly correct eating habits anywhere, by observing two rules only. The one is that the food shall not be of the refined variety, and the other that it must conform to known chemical requirements in the matter of combination with other foods eaten.

This ability allows the traveller to enjoy every country thoroughly, without the usual danger of strange foods. These people return from a world tour refreshed and invigorated, whereas before learning how to eat correctly they seldom travelled to foreign countries, and when they did so were compelled to restore their broken digestions after their return. Horace Fletcher once travelled to every civilized country and some uncivilized countries, and lived on the food of the natives, with not a moment of sickness, not even a cold or a headache, to mar his enjoyment of travel.

He had learned how to subsist on any food that is fit to eat, if this is natural enough to carry most of the elements with which nature originally endowed it, and if the laws of chemistry are observed in the combination of the various foods used.

One must know what constitutes a carbohydrate and what

a protein food, also what acid means in combination with starches.

Any carboyhdrate food is either starchy or sweet, and these require alkalin conditions for their complete digestion, so must not be combined with acids of any kind, as sour fruits, because the acid will neutralize the alkalin conditions necessary for the digestion of the starch or sugar.

Neither should these be combined with a protein of concentrated sort, such as meats, eggs, fish, or cheese, as these protein foods will excite too much hydrochloric acid during their stomach digestion, thus again taking away or neutralizing the alkalin conditions necessary for the digestion of the carbohydrates, the before-mentioned starches and sugars.

So one can still wreck the nutrition if observing the first requirement in regard to natural foods, but neglecting to observe the second, in regard to the correct chemical combination of the foods eaten.

If active, as a day laborer, or an athlete who is preparing for a contest, then the starches and sweets may be taken freely, as also the fats to a less extent; but the protein should remain at about the minimum for need in both classes.

One may eat at any modern hotel or restaurant and still not defy the conventional habit, by merely observing these three things; the natural character of the food as far as this may be possible, the correct separation of the incompatible foods mentioned above, and the proportioning of the foods of fuel character to the activities of the present.

Now let us see whether we can build three meals that will keep in mind these three indications outlined.

The breakfast for the active man may consist of three or four slices of whole wheat, rye or graham bread, well toasted or stale, not fresh; no acid fruits with this, so no orange juice or any other of the acid fruits, even though these may contain enough fruit sugar to give them a sweet taste; no meats, eggs, fish or cheese, as these will produce a high percentage of hydrochloric acid in the stomach, which would interfere with the alkalin conditions necessary for the digestion of the very starchy bread already selected. If coffee is taken habitually this may be allowed at this one meal, but should not be repeated during the day. Milk is not good with either the starches or the proteins, so is not recommended with the starchy bread. Sweet fruits, as dates, figs, or raisins, may be used with the bread, as these contain so much sugar and so little acid that they also require alkalin conditions for their digestion, even as the bread. Fat bacon, containing as it does so little protein, may be taken with the starchy breakfast; yolks of one or two eggs, containing not so very much protein, may also be admitted but are not recommended.

So the breakfast for the worker is limited to bread, with butter and honey if desired; a cup of coffee, with sugar if preferred, and with cream if this does not disagree; with this a dish of soaked dates, figs, or raisins, better not cooked, but dressed with cream. If this seems meager for the activities of the morning take it anyway for two or three weeks and you will find it ample; for you are not working on today's breakfast but on what you ate yesterday.

Breakfast for the sedentary person need not contain the bread, so will admit acid fruits nicely. A cup of coffee unsweetened, for those who must have it, together with a glassful of orange juice and a glass or two of milk, will make quite an ideal breakfast; but it will be better without the coffee.

Lunch for either class of occupation is best of nothing but vegetables, raw vegetable salads, fresh fruits and milk or buttermilk, with a soup if desired, but containing neither meat stock nor thickening, though the active subject may have butter or cream rather freely, while the sedentary should have very little fats of any kind.

The active person may again have the starches at noon, preferably in the form of lighter vegetable starches, as potatoes, but will have to pass up the acid fruits if starch is taken.

[156]

Dinner is really best eaten at the close of the day, and may be the heartiest meal of the day, containing the heaviest foods in the largest amounts, for night is approaching and sleep will offer opportunity for the complete digestion and metabolism of the foods eaten last; also there will be no physical or mental activities to detract from the disposal of the foods.

Many have the fixed habit of eating their principal meal of the day at noon. This is all right if only then there is keen desire for food. But the work of digestion requires a considerable amount of vitality, which will naturally detract from the vitality necessary for work; so we are less efficient either mentally or physically after a full meal than at other times.

The principal meal of the day for the active person may contain a fair serving of meat, eggs, fish, or cheese, as the piece de resistence, and also vegetables, raw salads, fresh fruits as freely as desired, thus offering foods that do not require alkalin conditions for their digestion. Since the meat or other concentrated protein requires much hydrochloric acid to activate the pepsin for the beginning of the protein digestion, it is evident that no carbohydrate food in concentrated form should be taken in conjunction with these proteins, as the carbohydrates, the starchy or sweet foods, require wholly alkalin conditions for their digestion, as you will not forget if you really wish to appropriate your food without the hampering fermentations that go with arrest of starchy digestion.

The active worker may indulge in starches twice a day, the sedentary one once a day or less; if in middle age or if very sedentary, it is safer to eschew the concentrated starches entirely, as such do not need the concentrated fuels that are so necessary for the active.

The evening meal may consist of a fruit cup or fruit cocktail, always unsweetened, of course, for sugar will not go with the acid digestion required by the protein; a soup made without meat stock or thickening, as meat soups represent plentiful amounts of the extractives of the meats, and it is better to eat the meat itself than to take the broth or soup from this; also the soup should not be thickened, as flour is used for this, and flour is a concentrated carbohydrate, and will not digest with the highly acid state of the gastric juice required for the meat or the other concentrated forms of protein; one fair serving of meat, eggs, fish, or cheese, baked, broiled, or roasted, but better not fried; cooked vegetables, such as beets, parsnips, turnips, carrots, spinach, chard, Brussels sprouts, cabbage, broccoli, roots or greens of every variety, excepting only the tubers, potatoes or winter squash, which contain too high a ratio of starch; raw vegetable salads of everything green that may be eaten raw, and dressed with oil and lemon, or sour cream, or oil mayonnaise if made without vinegar; all the fresh fruits desired, except banana, which contains twenty per cent carbohydrate, even as potato. Dessert may be a sliced fruit served with cream but no sugar, or a fruit gelatine, or a glass of fruit juices; and if coffee must be used see to it that this is unsweetened.

The active worker will take all these foods freely except the meat or other concentrated form of protein, of which he needs no more than does the sedentary; while the sedentary one will not require so much food of any kind except this same protein, which should be used in proportion to size of the eater, not in proportion to his activity.

Now that we have outlined three normal meals for those of different activity, let us put these in the form of a menu, for easy understanding of the thing.

It must be kept in mind that the whole menu is permitted, not required; so proportion the amounts to the real desire at the time, and do not try to eat the whole bill because it is offered; a mistake that is often made by those following suggested diets.

Never eat at all unless distinctly hungry; then eat only so much of even the right foods in the right way as keenly desired at the time.

[158]

CORRECT EATING HABITS

BREAKFAST

SEDENTARY

Glass or more of orange juice, or sliced acid fruit, with one or more glasses of milk. Fruit juice or fresh acid fruits are always to be unsweetened.

ACTIVE

Coffee if desired or very habitual, sweetened and creamed; three or four slices of toasted or stale whole wheat, rye or graham bread, well buttered and with honey, if desired; sliced fat bacon, broiled; a dish of soaked dates, figs or raisins.

LUNCH

SEDENTARY

Vegetable soup, without meat stock or thickening; cooked vegetables; raw salads, not dressed with vinegar; all the fresh fruit desired, except banana; a glass or two of milk or buttermilk; dessert of fruit ice, or sliced fruit, the latter unsweetened, and the fruit ice not ideal because sweetened.

ACTIVE

Vegetable soup without stock or thickening; raw vegetable salads, dressed without vinegar or other acid dressing, but plain oil or sour cream; cooked vegetables of all kinds; baked potato or toasted whole wheat bread, if very active; sweet fruits, as dates, figs or raisins, with honey and cream, or a dish of ice cream; if coffee must be used, this also may contain both sugar and cream, but it is better not to form the coffee habit.

DINNER

SEDENTARY

Vegetable soup if desired, but without stock or thickening; raw vegetable salads of all available vegetables, roots or greens, dressed with oil and lemon juice, or with plain sour cream, but no vinegar; all the cooked vegetables desired, with oil or lemon dressing, or butter if used moderately; one moderate serving

ACTIVE

Any soup without meat stock or thickening; as many cooked vegetables as desired, no starchy tubers, as potato or winter squash; large raw vegetable salads of anything available, even cabbage, if nothing more can be readily obtained, dressed with lemon juice and oil or with plain sour cream; one fair serving

[159]

of meat, eggs, fish or cheese; sliced fruit dessert, or fruited gelatine, unsweetened; if coffee must be used, then always unsweetened.

of meat, eggs, fish, or cheese; sliced fruits or fruited gelatine, always unsweetened; if coffee must be used be sure this is unsweetened.

Children come under the active group, and may have the same foods as the active adult, for their much greater activity calls for more fuel foods than are good for the sedentary adult.

Ill children should have no other foods than fruit juices or fresh fruits till well, which does not take long if so fed.

CHAPTER XIV.

The Banqueting Habit

W E have grown into a nation of banqueters through accompanying every function with the eating of foods of huge variety and infernal potency for harm.

It is difficult to get out an audience for any function that is not associated in some way with eating. Even church functions, in which religious fervor should be incentive enough for attendance of the faithful, are meagerly attended if the ladies do not provide at the same time a feast for the audience.

The conditions resulting from the too frequent and free use of those foods that appear at public banquets are best described, perhaps, as "congressman's disease," the thing the late Senator Tillman, of South Carolina, charged to the usual habit of banqueting that attends sessions of the national congress.

When a congressman dedicates a new federal building, or is the speaker at some function of sufficient scope to warrant the appearance of a congressman or senator, he is subjected to a banquet, or a series of banquets, with the result that he is incapacitated too often through overeating. It was this to which Senator Tillman charged his own breakdown at sixty-three years of age, when he suffered a stroke of apoplexy and dropped on the Capitol steps.

He restored his health through abstemious eating of the right foods; and when again representing his state in the senate he became known as the "health mentor of the senate" through his frequent warnings to his fellow senators that there were many of them going the same way as he, through the use of too rich foods in too great and too frequent amounts.

Admiral Togo, of Japan, when visiting in this country a number of years before the World War, was compelled to cut short his intended stay on account of the frequency with which he was forced to appear at banquets. He said the American people were a nation of banqueters, and his health forbade his indulging in such frequent eating of banquet fare.

We have lost sight of the true function of foods when we make eating any part of a social function; for food is replacement material only, nothing more; and when we need replacement of body tissues or body fuels then we need food, and at no other time.

Why can we not have our social functions wholly apart from the taking of nourishment? Eating is serious business, and if intelligently administered it is restorative, constructive; while if poorly administered it is far more destructive than the whiskey habit.

There is no investment in time or thought or care that will pay nearly so large dividends as the study of body needs in the matter of food.

To supply the body with just what is needed, to avoid the usual excesses in food, to make sure that when food is really required we do not flout the immutable laws of chemistry in our combination of food elements — these things are a vital consideration in our every day living.

If we are properly nourished we are never tired, never sick, never discouraged or subject to blues; we are optimistic, cheerful, capable; we think clearly, make our decisions quickly and correctly; we have ambition and stick-to-itiveness, all attributes of health; while if we administer diet improperly we are the reverse of all this, and we suffer from inefficiency to a shocking degree.

This difference is chargeable directly to the state of our nutrition at the time, and nutrition is directly the result of what we eat and how we eat.

Does this not make of eating a serious business?

There is no reason why the banquet cannot be indulged in within certain limits, if the menu is proper, and if the meal does not represent extra and unneeded nourishment.

There is a line of eating "joints" whose slogan is: "That

Extra Bite;" and it is just that extra bite that does so much harm in most cases. When we have eaten sufficiently at meals to satisfy immediate desire, we never need that extra bite, nor should we ever have it.

The habit of eating between meals is potent with harm, for not only do we get through this habit much unneeded nourishment, but we thoroughly destroy what might easily be cultivated into a correct habit of eating; and soon we do not actually know when we are hungry, having at all times a sort of desire to eat something, to take a little nourishment.

I have often observed young men who were normally active, who were apparently well, often athletic, who could be found in some eating place between meals almost any day, often three or more times each day, eating a piece of pie and a glass of milk or a cup of coffee, or a sandwich and a cup of coffee, and in every case the athletic career of such was short, and it was not long till disease in some form was in evidence.

One such young man, the pitcher for the local ball team, could be counted on to sit in at the local restaurant at least three times a day for an extra bite, though he was an abnormally heavy eater at home three times a day.

His family were contributors to the writer's budget; and as the family table habits were full and free they were naturally heavy contributors. But this one young man was such an irrational eater that he was warned that his usefulness to the ball team or even to his family would be short lived unless he ate less and was more careful as to what he ate. He would not listen, of course, for he felt all right, though often he was too tired to work, and occasionally pitched a poor game for the same reason.

At twenty years of age he developed rheumatism; he suffered involvement of the lining of the heart, endocarditis, which crippled his heart valves; and from being a young fellow of tremendous strength, noted for his feats of all kinds, he became a complete invalid at twenty-two, and never again was

[163]

able to indulge in athletics or even to earn a living at work of any kind.

He banqueted three times a day at home, and three or more times a day he had that extra bite which he could not be persuaded that he did not need.

When a young man glorying in his strength is told that his way of living is soon going to cut short his athletic ability, even to ruin his health, he will not listen, for he cannot imagine anything that could get him; yet he is laying the foundation for early breakdown when he eats three large meals a day of poorly selected and incorrectly combined foods; and when he adds to this the further handicap of that extra bite three times a day, he is asking of a splendid body more than it can be expected to perform.

When the writer was fifty years of age he made a hunting trip of eight or more hours of hard walking and severe hill climbing with the young pitcher before referred to, on a rabbit hunt.

We met at the train and headed straight for the woods, at nine-thirty in the morning.

His first greeting was: "What did you have for breakfast, Doc?"

He was told that breakfast for the writer occurred about five or five-thirty P.M. George remarked that this was a man's hike, and it would be too bad to wait all day for a man who was too weak to walk the rugged hills over which we planned our hunt.

My question was: "What did you have, George?" His companion was eighteen years of age, the catcher for the ball team, and George turned to Bill and said, "What did we have, Bill?" Between them they figured a breakfast that represented two bowls of oatmeal, 20 or more buckwheat pancakes, butter and maple syrup, sausage galore, three or four slices each of bread (presumably the usual white variety), three or four doughnuts, and there was a dispute as to whether the pancakes numbered

20 or more apiece, for they said they ate them as fast as Bill's mother could bake them; each had had two cups of coffee also.

A man's breakfast, for a man's hike, as George explained it.

At eleven o'clock Bill complained of being hungry, but George said if they ate then they would be so weak they could not continue the hunt till dark, as planned, so refused to spread the lunch; but a half hour later Bill sat down on a log and refused to go any farther till he had been fed, as he said he was too weak to walk farther.

Grumbling, George set out his lunch, consisting of a chunk of cheese of near a pound, a dozen sandwiches, a dozen doughnuts, and two bars of chocolate. They invited me to join them, but I refused, as there was no sign as yet of hunger. One of the dogs would follow me, so he was taken out while the boys ate, and in a half hour a return to the feeding log showed the boys ready to go.

Bill did not hunt any more that day, as he was too tired, and complained that one knee was no good; but George stuck to the hunt till it was so dark that only the white tail of a rabbit could be seen dancing out of sight. As his bag and mine were loaded to the limit we decided to call it a day. Bill had moved from log to log all afternoon and waited till the hunt again came his way, but had only the three rabbits which he had shot before eleven-thirty.

George was too tired to carry his gun, so withdrew the shells and dragged it by the muzzle the quarter of a mile from the woods across the valley to his house, where we were to eat supper.

When he entered the house he dropped his heavy hunting coat containing his ten rabbits on the floor, also his gun, threw himself on a divan with a groan, and went at once into a heavy sleep. Bill did not stop, but went on to his own house, where he said he was going to bed.

The writer sang songs with a younger brother of George till supper was called, then resumed singing till train time, and left for home with no sense of weariness whatever, simply because he was not laboring with a heavy digestive task while hunting. The two boys had a man's work to do in digesting so much heavy food, without the fatiguing walking over hilly country, climbing steep hills all day, and putting in perhaps eight hours of real work of this strenuous sort.

Ten rabbits will weigh close to thirty pounds, which is in itself a considerable handicap when carried for hours; and this, with the continual alertness necessary in quick shooting of aimlessly scooting rabbits, is a considerable tax on endurance; yet there was no sense of weariness at all, rather an exhiliration from the day in the woods.

Bill died a hero in the late war, while George developed rheumatism soon after this day in the woods, and never again was himself.

Ten years before this the writer had been a banqueter, and had eaten himself into a state of utter uselessness. It was after these ten years of sensible eating that he was able to outdo these two young men of eighteen and twenty years who were notably strong and in the full flush of youthful enthusiasm, presumably, but both handicapped by such a fatigue as can come from nothing else than from badly administered eating habits.

Few realize what a sense of weariness is costing them every day or they would be more careful in avoiding this universal cause of all fatigue.

To go on and on, hour after hour all day long, without any hampering sense of weariness, is worth more than a sizable legacy; and this is possible to anyone who will avoid the usual dietary mistakes and give to the subject of eating at least as much care and attention as he would devote to any ordinary business problem.

There is a very good way to change eating habits, and that is to stop eating till appetite leaves.

To stop suddenly from eating anything at all is to go through a very distressing period of weakness, faintness, and gnawing hunger; so few are willing to undertake this, as the missing of one meal is so very disagreeable.

The best way to approach the fast is to miss one meal a day for a time, then two meals, then drop the third meal, till food soon loses its imminent significance, and becomes something remote in thought.

It is verily a surprise to anyone who has never undertaken to stop eating for a time, that after two or three days wholly without food there is no appetite at all; and one wonders why he ever thought it so vitally important that he eat three meals every day, or six meals, which is not uncommon.

A part of what we eat is stored as fuel for emergencies that may arise later, such stores representing fats, glycogens and free albumens, all available for food when no outer supply is available. To fast for thirty to sixty days is by no means an uncommon thing today, while in early times the fast was the usual mode of correcting bodily ailments.

Surely if our troubles come from stored and circulating toxins then the fast is a normal way of correcting this wrong condition.

To fast when in full health is not considered reasonable; but there have been those who never waited till sickness developed, but who fasted at certain fixed times each year, or several times a year, for the simple reason that following each such fast was a period of regeneration that was most refreshing indeed, and life was always lived on a much higher plane than before.

Banqueting when in seeming health is common, and nothing is thought of frequent eating without apparent need of food; but even this practice is not half so reprehensible as the universal habit of feeding the sick.

Surely when illness is present and no appetite is in evidence, it is something little short of insanity that would suggest food of any kind. There is not an animal known that will eat

[167]

anything when less than well, even the lowly hog stubbornly refusing food when really ill.

Man alone seems to think that he is compelled to "eat to keep up his strength" whether well or ill.

Eating not wisely but much too well is causing most of our illnesses, and the same thing keeps them up. Yet it is so simple and easy to eat only when really hungry, and to absolutely refuse all food when not hungry, that it is a wonder that such a mistaken habit ever could have developed as eating when not hungry, and especially taking "something" when the thought of all food is even repugnant to one.

Yet the average doctor and the average hospital will insist on nourishment in some form no matter how ill the subject may be, under the seeming impression that dire calamity will follow if meals are missed.

Is man more intelligent than his little brothers, and should the ill be fed whether or not they wish food?

The cat or dog when ill lies and sleeps most of the time, refusing all food, and when allowed to pursue its own instinct seldom fails to recover in a short time. But man, the supreme intelligence of the earth, who looks down on the unintelligence of the little furry or feathered brothers as incapable of reasoning, is up against it when ill; for he feels that nature is not to be read literally in the matter of food, and still seems to believe that his own boasted intelligence is a better guide than nature which created him and keeps him going.

Desire always points the way to need, and it is only so that nature keeps all her children out of trouble. But when desire has been so corrected and subjected to conventional restrictions and limitations it does cease to be a correct guide.

Better fast for a time every few months or every year, till the habit appetites are thoroughly broken; then begin by eating only when hungry, of the natural foods, combining these compatibly, and note the change this makes in bodily condition and one's whole outlook on life.

Epileptics have fasted for a month and never again suffered a return of the convulsions. Nephritis, diabetes, skin diseases, asthma, all recover in the absence of all food; also all other diseases that result from wrong chemistry will readjust themselves when the body is free to give all its attention to cleaning house.

An attorney in Buffalo who was suffering from diabetes for a number of years, and whose mental condition was such that his friends were all pitying him, went to his cottage in central Canada for a few weeks of rest, and decided to walk around the head of the lake to a store three or four miles distant.

He had no difficulty in finding the store, but his return was beset by branching trails that made it difficult to know which was the way to his cottage. The result was that he was lost for twelve days in unfamiliar woods, far from any trail; and when the other cottagers organized a searching party and finally located him, expecting to find him dead, they were surprised to see him active and feeling fine, but so much thinner that they thought he must be starving.

In this one experience he learned that after the first two or three days of fasting there is no hunger in evidence, and the body begins to feed on its stores. He never showed sugar again in his urine, for he never again overate, as was his custom before he became lost.

So he said he did not regret having been lost for twelve days so long as he lost his diabetes and found that it stayed lost.

He resumed his practice and found that his head was all right, which is sure to be the case when the body is right.

Cases who are lost in the woods and found dead after as short periods as twelve days, as has occurred many times, have died through fright, not starvation; for the body in ordinary flesh will subsist nicely for thirty days or more with nothing at all.

It is different when at sea in an open boat, for the heat

or cold of continuous exposure, together with the inability to get water, will not infrequently terminate life in ten or twelve days; and yet it is not at all unlikely that even in this case fright plays a great part.

Six years ago in Buffalo a little cat, not yet full grown, was chased up a tree to a housetop, where its cries were not heard. For thirty days it lived there without food, and possibly with little water, except as rain might have left water within reach. When discovered by a boy who was climbing a telephone pole nearby, and finally rescued, it was in good condition and very lively, but thin to the point of extreme emaciation. Its absence had been noted thirty days before, and its mistress had given it up as lost; but all this time it had been fasting on her own roof.

The hibernating animals fast for ninety days or more, and always without harm. They do not have any special arrangement by which nature permits of this long fast, for any animal could do the same, yet no more than can man.

Banqueting consists of eating unneeded food, whether this be in public or private; and feeding in illness is banqueting.

If nothing more could be done for the ill than to let them severely alone, the death rates would decline markedly.

If disease has slain its thousands, then feeding in illness has slain its tens of thousands, and is a wanton waste of life.

If you must be present at an evening banquet, then at least eat nothing at dinner preceding this, or at most, nothing but orange juice; then at the banquet table leave out the most incompatible foods served, or decide whether you will take the starchy things or the proteins. But do not, as you value your future health, take the entire bill as most banqueters do, even complaining sometimes that the bill was not wide enough, high enough, or deep enough for their desires.

CHAPTER XV.

Exercise

NO book that purports to teach the ways of health should omit exercise, of course; but we will not attempt here to put forth a system of exercises, as there are so many extant, all of which are good. The philosophy of exercise will occupy all our attention, leaving the various systems to suggest themselves, or counting on the restored vitality that comes through correct eating to point the way to all exercise.

It is through exercise that we develop, and if we were continually inert we would never develop properly.

The more any muscle is exercised the better does it function, with one restriction, and that is fatigue.

Exercise below the point of fatigue leads to development of the organ or tissue exercised; beyond fatigue it leads to deterioration.

Nature uses the sense of fatigue to tell us when we have gone far enough for the time and need rest; to drive the body on and on after the warning of fatigue has been felt is to invite deterioration of function, instead of development.

Through the sense of hunger nature tells us when we need food; through the sense of thirst she tells us when we need more fluids; and through the sense of fatigue she tells us when we need rest; so we must heed all of her warnings if we would assist her to keep us as well as she intends us to be.

The one who is driving himself day after day against a sense of weariness that is all but over-powering is headed straight for an early breakdown.

There are those who are never anything but tired, and who cannot do anything without this sense of weariness. Such a person is sick, whether or not this is realized, and should clean house and so arrange the dietary habit as to stop the manufacture of the end-products of digestion and metabolism that alone causes this sense of weariness. Till this is done there is no use in prescribing exercise; for the aggravation of this sense of weariness will arrest digestion, absorption, and metabolism, largely, and do vast harm.

There have been cases restored through prescribed and forced exercise, but at considerable risk; for such might and usually do break down through inadvisable attempts to get well in this way.

First relieve the cause of the weariness and then exercise will be taken voluntarily, for it is impossible to restrain the desire to take active exercise when one is as well as one should be.

After all, exercise is a great help in restoring the body to a better condition, but only in the absence of this weariness that makes of the effort to exercise something to be dreaded.

When we sleep we breathe far deeper than when waking, as it is during sleep that we oxidize our waste matter and eliminate much of this through the lungs. What we do while sleeping we can do also when awake through exercise, by the forced respiration and the free perspiration that accompany exercise of sufficient violence to compel both.

The mild exercises of the morning daily dozen are of some use, but cannot be compared to those supplied through games of any sort that demand strenuous exertion.

The more muscles we use, and the larger the groups brought into play, the more do we speed up both respiration and circulation of the blood. If the exercises are strenuous enough and continued long enough the pores of the skin also are brought into exalted action, and we eliminate in perspiration much toxic material that under less strenuous exercise would be compelled to find its way out through other of the eliminative channels or fail of elimination.

Running and swimming are for this reason ideal exercises, as both call into play the larger groups of muscles.

Rowing is excellent for the same reason, as well as because of the continual massage of the abdominal organs, gained by bending and pulling.

The benefits of exercise are through this massage of the muscles themselves and of the internal organs, as of course through increased respiration, circulation and perspiration.

It is through oxidation of the contained glycogen stored in the muscular tissue that we generate power, and the faster this is used up the sooner will we have to replace this through glycogen-building foods, such as starches and sugars; so the more active exercise we take the more of these carbohydrate foods can we consume without harm.

This is why the sedentary person should not try to live on the same foods or the same amounts as the active man, for an excess of carbonaceous or fuel foods acts just the same in a man as a too rich mixture of gases acts in the motor, resulting in the deposit of carbon.

We do not wear out, as a rule, but we rust out; or we clog ourselves with the debris of combustion, and we become carboned just as does the gasoline motor.

If we never think, how in the name of common sense can we expect to develop mentality? Similarly, if we never use our muscles, how can we expect to develop these?

Every organ of the body is used every day, hence it develops; and without this use it would never develop; for nature does not for long perpetuate a useless function of any kind.

If we keep one rule in mind we will do well when we seek to develop through exercise; and that rule is that all exercise below the point of fatigue is beneficial, highly so, while beyond the fatigue point exercise is harmful, increasing our toxic state because it is creating more debris for a system already badly overloaded with this very substance.

The heart develops enormous power, and through its frequent contractions it develops foot-pounds of energy daily that would stagger one to believe.

[173]

Yet the heart rests, nearly or quite three-fifths of the time, for it works only two-fifths of the time, or that represented' by its contraction; the period of relaxation, while it is filling with blood for the next systole, is one of rest, or passivity.

The respiratory muscles do not work all the time, for it is only during inspiration that they are active, expiration being a period of passivity for the respiratory muscles, when the weight of the chest and the elasticity of the tissues force out the air, wholly without muscular effort of any degree, except during active exercise, when our need for air is so great that we cannot wait for passive expiration but must hurry this by a muscular effort, in order to get the next breath quickly.

The muscular movements of the digestive tract are not continuous, for it is only during active digestion that the peristaltic waves, or muscular contractions occur, and in the intervals of their movements there is rest, perhaps equal to the period of contraction.

So no part of the body works continuously, as we so often think it does; and the law of exercise and rest is observed in all our body functions, else they could never continue to be efficient.

As with each part, even so with the whole man; for he cannot work all the time, if he would keep in good condition. He must have rest in order to recuperate from the work of oxidation that he has compelled by his exercise.

This is what sleep is for, to allow us time to work over the material taken in through the day, oxidize or burn up the waste products and get them ready for elimination.

Eight hours of work, eight hours of recreation and eight hours of sleep is a fair division of the days and life-time days for everyone, and it is not well to try to cut short any one of these periods.

We need work, exercise, play, rest, all of which help us to keep clean inside, and to enjoy all these periods as only one can do who is giving to each its due meed.

If we work too long or too hard it spoils our recreation, and it too often spoils our sleep; for it is not infrequently that we feel too tired to sleep well.

If we give too much time to recreation we sicken of this, and then it is not long till everything palls on us, and we cannot find anything to amuse us.

If we work hard and faithfully for eight hours, then our recreation is far more thoroughly enjoyed, and our sleep will be more refreshing.

The sedentary individual needs some very active exercise every day to offset the lack of oxidation necessitated by sedentary work, for it is well, it is almost necessary, to do something every day to speed up our motor, force the draught, shake the grates, in order to make our fires burn more brightly.

To be without exercise is to become stagnant, like the stream without current; and how we do load up with waste if stagnant!

When one cultivates the habit of eating only so much as is really needed, and at the same time keeps very active, he insures the full oxidation of his debris, and he will be surprised after a few months to discover that he is consuming less food than when formerly inactive.

The life of the average athlete is greatly shortened by his food habits, as well as by his too strenuous exercise, and usually this is chiefly through his food habits.

To develop a great need for food through strenuous exercise, and then to settle down into a sedentary occupation, as the college athlete so frequently does, is to invite disaster within a few years, unless the food habits are changed to fit the sedentary life, a thing that is too often neglected till after the breakdown occurs.

A training table appetite is too often carried into sedentary life, and wrecks the machine far faster than if these habits are continued and the customary exercises kept up faithfully; so if you are on a training diet you must never quit training;

or if you quit training then the training table habit of eating must at once be cut off.

We can increase endurance through exercise, of course; for the more of our fuels we burn up and eliminate, the more readily do we consume the new supply and the sooner do we remove the ashes of activity.

Endurance consists in the thorough removal, the prompt and complete removal, of all debris created in the used area by our exercise. If these ashes of activity can be removed quickly, then there is opportunity for more combustion to create more energy; but if the ashes remain largely in the field of activity, the used muscle becomes clogged with it and the nerve spark will not easily ignite the next charge of fuel for the next effort, and the muscle tires, that is, it cannot get the necessary energy for further effort.

Now it is easy to see that energy, being derived from the combustion of fuels in the muscles employed, cannot continue to develop without interruption unless all the conditions necessary for this are present.

If the tissues are laden with the ashes of former combustion, it is not difficult to see that no very great energy can be developed here; for combustion depends on the union of oxygen with the fuel, ignited by an impulse in the form of the nerve spark.

It is exactly the same as any fire that develops heat or power; for unless its ashes are kept removed these will smother the fire and there will be little heat.

So unless the tissues are fairly clear of waste there is difficult oxidation of the fuels and little energy; and the longer the effort, the more waste will be created and the greater will be the accumulation of debris.

Endurance requires a clean field for operation, therefore little of the acid end-products, the fatigue poisons.

By every consideration of disease do we find that cleanliness stands first as a preventive. Our former diseases of filth, such as typhoid or typhus fever, smallpox, yellow fever, malaria, are dying out with each generation, not through supposed applied immunization, but merely because sanitary engineers have learned that accumulation of debris is back of all filth diseases, and have devised means for perfect sewerage, drainage and combustion of debris that in the earlier days scourged London and other cities with decimating filth diseases year after year.

London was a festering sore among the more civilized nations, in the early days, when smallpox, plague, decimated the population year after year. At that time London had no sewer system, and the gutters of the streets ran foul with sewage, while the stench was such that the more aesthetic of the population stayed indoors with the windows closed to shut out the odors.

About the time London developed a system of sewerage, Jenner discovered the supposed relation between smallpox and cowpox. From the smallpox (so-called) on the cow's udder he constructed what he called a vaccine, which was introduced under the skin of the healthy, or the so-called healthy, which was supposed to render the vaccinated immune to smallpox throughout life.

He vaccinated his own son, who a few years later died of tuberculosis, and by persuasion he brought many of the medical profession to believe that his newly discovered theory of immunity through vaccination of the uninfected with cowpox was a vastly safer proceeding than the usual custom then in vogue of arm to arm inoculation.

As other physicians began to practice the same methods there was a feeling that this was the way out of the scourge of smallpox. Arm to arm inoculation had taken such fearful toll of life that soon Parliament was persuaded to reward Jenner with thirty thousand pounds for his discovery, and to endorse vaccination and forbid the former arm to arm inocu-

[177]

lation; and vaccination became the recognized form of supposed prevention for smallpox.

This was about one hundred and thirty-five years ago, and till 1870 vaccination was entirely compulsory in England, every infant being subjected to the heathen rite of vaccination, and smallpox began to decline throughout all England.

But sanitation had been born about this time, and London, the seat and center of smallpox, began to cash in on the improved health conditions resulting from this real discovery, while vaccination took the credit.

After 1870 the vaccination laws began to be less rigidly enforced, and by 1898 a conscience clause was adopted that permitted the easement of the law to omit vaccination in those who for any reason were conscientiously opposed to its application to their own persons or those of their families. Vaccination since that time has steadily declined in England, till today it is probable that far less than half of the population has been vaccinated at all. Yet smallpox has continued to decline in England till today it is one of the lowest in vital statistics, as these relate to smallpox incidence or smallpox mortality.

Also, those nations thoroughly vaccinated, as the Philippine Islands, Japan, Italy, have today the highest incidence and the highest mortality from smallpox of all nations, while those nations that do not observe the rite of vaccination are lowest in both morbidity and mortality.

If vaccination prevents smallpox, then those nations enforcing vaccination should be free from the plague, and those who neglect this rite should suffer heavy penalty for this. Yet the opposite is true, as anyone can prove by consulting the vital statistics of every civilized country keeping health records.

Now all this has no apparent connection with exercise, but it is actually closely related to the whole subject of keeping clean inside; and what keeps the whole man clean inside prevents disease, just as what keeps the community clean and sanitary prevents the diseases that result from filth.

Smallpox is a type of filth disease, and is controlled only through sanitation, never through vaccination; and sanitation means the removal of accumulating filth.

Personal sanitation means exactly the same thing as regards the individual; for when we do not accumulate waste or filth internally we do not have disease, and exercise helps mightily to remove waste matter of all kinds through the heightened oxidation resulting from the increase of circulation and respiration, as well as through elimination directly through the skin by perspiration.

As the filth diseases have declined through better understanding of the laws of sanitation, just so will the personal disease decline through application of exactly the same principles to the individual body.

It is necessary to learn how to create less acid end-products from foods and metabolism of foods, and it is scarcely less necessary to learn the very direct connection between activity or its opposite and the state of the tissues.

Many will fear to take active exercise after forty years of age, lest the heart be damaged. To make sure that the heart will not be damaged, it is best to clean house first, then adopt habits of diet that will not create again such vast amounts of the acid end-products as are the rule. Exercise gently at first, then increase the effort continually till a heart that may formerly have been less than competent for strenuous exercise will develop a capability for the most strenuous of sports, even tennis, the most fatiguing of all games after rowing.

Dr. Anderson, formerly physical director at Yale, classified the sports of college in the order of their demand on vitality, and he placed the four mile rowing stunt first, as requiring the greatest amount of stamina, and tennis second, even ahead of the mile run and the football and track sports, even handball, which is considered one of the most strenuous sports.

The most successful man in restoring hearts was Oertel, of Switzerland, and we have for years recognized the Oertel plan of heart treatment as being applicable to many types of heart disease.

Oertel had his patients with weak hearts start climbing the nearest peak of the Alps, always stopping when the breathing became at all labored. Each day the patient tried his climb, and soon discovered that each day he could climb a step or two further before distress was in evidence; and so by progressive exercise of the heart, strength of this weakened muscle was developed.

Milo, the fabled Greek, was supposed to have carried a small calf every day around the stadium of Athens; and as the calf grew, so did Milo's ability to carry it, till when it was a bull Milo could still carry it around the stadium track.

The most successful systems of strength development are founded on exactly the same principle, one of graduated exercises; and fatigue is to be avoided if the development is to progress satisfactorily.

If you can lift one hundred pounds over your head you are a fairly strong man; but it would not be good to do this every day if the task required your full strength. Rather set the task at not more than three quarters of the full strength or capacity, and repeat till fatigue shows mildly; and if you persist in this test every day or every other day you will soon find that your strength has increased so that you can add several pounds and still perform your task easily.

If you use weights for exercise always proportion the task to a half or not more than three quarters of your present capacity, and you will then be able to increase your strength and endurance.

CHAPTER XVI.

The Psychology of Health

WHAT effect does thinking have on health, and what effect has proper health on thinking?

In a former chapter we discussed the effect of food on the mind, and there we stated that food has a very direct effect on the mind, even more pronounced than on bodily health, in many cases. In all cases there is a liberating effect on thought when the body is freed through correct eating habit, from the depressing effects of the acid end-products of digestion and metabolism.

Man is a trinity, spiritual, mental, physical; and if it is true that the bodily condition is reflected on the state of mind and thought, it is equally true, it must be true, the other way around.

We know that the body can be ruined through mental stresses, if these are sufficiently severe to interfere with normal function, as they easily can do.

Fright has turned the hair white in a night; it has also killed, by interference with normal function.

If great stresses can so influence the body, then it is fair to suppose that stresses of less degree have a depressing effect on function during their persistence.

Thus living with a depressing thought can gradually wreck the finest body, through continually depressing function to some degree.

Fatigue, if continued day after day, is depressing to function of every sort, as is also grief, worry, fear, sorrow, suspicion, jealousy.

Defeat is deadly; and if we accept it, we are losers by a far greater degree than we can realize.

If we take the attitude that "the harder you fall the higher you bounce"; if we use each set-back as a new starting point;

if we refuse stubbornly to accept defeat, but rather start in
to struggle harder than ever for success, there is no combination of circumstances that can put us down to stay.

"It isn't whether you win, my son, but only HOW DID
YOU FIGHT?"

Nothing will so subjugate the will and desire for health as
continued fatigue; and nothing so robs the psychology of a
punch as this very same thing.

All the preaching of the psychologist, and all of his en-
couragement to pick one's self up and try again, have little effect on the tired subject, for he gradually comes to accept a
defeatist attitude, and feels that the entire world is arrayed
against him.

If we can get the idea that all of our ailments, fatigue,
disease, old age, death itself, come from an inability of the
body to keep itself clear of its own irritating acid end-products
of digestion and metabolism, to keep itself clean, in other
words, then we will see that we are under great necessity of
keeping the tissues clear of this debris continually; and we will
soon cease to crave or expect sympathy for our ills, knowing
that they are all self-created, that no one is to blame for our
condition except ourselves.

This in itself is a psychology greatly to be desired, and
makes of our condition anything we wish it to be, IF we have
the will power, the understanding, and the determination to accomplish such a change in our physical and mental health as
is always possible to anyone.

Nature plays no favorites; she treats her children all exactly
alike; and the difference in condition is due either to self-in-
flicted causes, or is inherited from misunderstanding parents,
or is forced on us by fortuitous circumstances that may have
been beyond our control.

In any case if we accept the attitude of defeat we are lost;
we are in the way of those who may fill our places better; and
we would do well to accept the facts as either of our own

creating, or make the best of what inheritance we have and fight to better this.

Every day the sun rises, whether we see it or not, and every day it will continue to rise till the end of the world. Each day is a new day, the old is past and buried, never to be again lived over or through.

The water that has passed under the bridge is gone forever and we will never grind our grist with that; but it still flows; and each day the supply is sufficient for our grinding; so forget the water that has passed, and grind effectively with what is still available.

What if we have failed to accomplish today what we aimed at yesterday? Tomorrow is another and brand new day, filled with all the opportunities for success that any day can offer; so let us close today's book and start in on tomorrow's chances, forgetting completely past failures.

If we have failed today to realize the control of the body we had promised ourselves for today, why, tomorrow is just around the corner, and we can make of every failure a guide for tomorrow's success.

If we have tried for months to achieve health without any apparent gain, remember that the body grows little by little, that it dies little by little, and is replaced little by little with new cells; so as long as this spirit of growth persists, which is as long as life lasts, we are facing tomorrows and tomorrows, each with its opportunities for improvement, and we shall surely reap the full reward if we do not give up the fight.

It is a most comforting thought that we are dying daily and daily being reborn, cell by cell; and that so long as we are in control of what goes into us, just so long can we determine of what materials we will construct the new body.

No one can eat our food for us; no one can wholly dictate the selection of our foods, unless we are boarding at the usual boarding house; no one can digest our food but us; no one can absorb it, assimilate it, metabolize it, excrete the waste from it,

but us; so the rebuilding of our bodies daily is up to us, and
to no one else in the whole world.

This, then, is a matter under our own control, surely, and
when we are less than well who is to blame except ourselves?

This takes fatigue, disease, old age and death itself out of
the class of pitiable conditions, however pitiful they seem, and
charges us each with the entire responsibility for our own condition daily, throughout life, after we have reached the age
of self-control and are no longer dependent on the guidance
of parents who may wholly misunderstand the things that pertain to bodily function.

If we have allowed appetite to control our selection of food
instead of determining what is the particular need of the body;
if we have overeaten; if we have gotten drunk with food, or
alcoholic beverages; if we have eaten not wisely but too well,
against our better judgement; — if we have failed, in other
words, to be guided by the instinct in food selection that will
safeguard our nutrition continually, why, today is but today,
and tomorrow offers opportunity to correct the thing through
these very mistakes. We can remember that the body today
is not wholly the body of tomorrow; that some of its parts or
cells have died in the night and new cells have been born; so
we can start from this point and make of the coming day one
of regeneration instead of degeneration.

The preponderance of regenerative days over degenerative
days determines ultimate regeneration instead of its opposite.
We have the decision within our power as to whether we
will live regeneratively or degeneratively; and no one should
be allowed to influence us in the least in our decision, for we
alone are the mentors of ourselves and our condition.

When one begins to live differently from the mob, when the
life departs from the conventional mob plan in any degree or
any particular, then it is that criticism starts; and this is most
disconcerting to one who is easily influenced by mob thought,
or who reveres the opinions of others above his own.

[184]

After observing the reactions of returning health in many thousands of cases during the past twenty-six years, it is still somewhat surprising to see the complete change in psychology that sets in very soon after the way is opened for regeneration of function.

To adopt the regenerative plan of eating is to invite chemical changes in the body that result in a complete rearrangement of the whole man; and the very first step is the loss of weight, as the body begins to throw off the waste matter long carried.

To one who has husbanded every pound most carefully for years on account of habitual lightness of weight, this loss is rather disconcerting, surely; but such must realize that the body cannot keep all the old materials and at the same time completely change its chemistry; so this loss of weight must be looked on as merely a part of the housecleaning program now setting in, getting rid of the old in order to properly create an ideal new.

To offset this seemingly disastrous loss of weight there is a change in the psychology that almost compels a realization of this very fact; and however the friends may clamor and predict dire results, it is rather infrequently that the one well-launched on a regenerative plan of eating will turn back.

There are of course those timid souls that fear everything, to whom every opinion of friends, family or physician has more weight than their own powers of reasoning, and who see ahead all the dreadful possibilities predicted by those who do not understand, and finally turn back. But they are few in comparison to those who have felt the subtle changes that indicate improving condition, and who can shut eyes and ears to the calamitous predictions of others and keep right on to the goal that means better health than ever before, more accomplishment, better work, more enjoyment in work and even in living, yes, even in eating, than was the rule before.

Such may look under par for one or two years, before the

body has sufficiently changed its abnormal chemistry to the more normal; and all this time friends will be clamorous against the foolish idea of dieting. But in the end, when the body is sufficiently changed to insure far better function in every way, even the appearance is so improved that no more jibes or friendly warnings are heard, only exclamations over how well one looks; yet this experience has little or no effect on the friends or family, for by this time they have forgotten the former ill health of the subject and think the improvement merely one of those things that happen.

The writer has seen many of these reborn subjects return to the very same physicians who formerly had condemned these self-same cases to early demise, following continually degenerating conditions, but he has yet to find one who accepted the truth of a self-conducted regeneration, all regarding such cases as merely "another of those things."

Health has its own psychology, in no wise related to that of ill health; and once having experienced this uplifting psychology, few are willing to give it up and return to the indiscriminate eating of all sorts of heterogeneous mixtures of incompatible and inimical foods that forms the usual habit of the average man or woman.

More failures result from wrong bodily condition than from fortuitous aberrations of the stock market; for the resulting psychology is one of defeat when the body is not at par, or better than the average body; and the mind is poorly supported when its circulation is laden with all sorts of irritating acid end-products.

If this is true, then it is equally true that a mind supported by a proper blood chemistry is in better position to cope with whatever happens than is one punished with debris; and so it is.

Instances are numerous in which several people banded together to impress on someone else the idea that he was not well; and in every case there is a response to these adverse suggestions that sometimes does result in actual illness, surely in such an idea of illness that it is laughable that the victim could be so gullible.

Everyone is subject to adverse suggestion, to a greater or less degree, though it is possible that not everyone could be made actually ill by being continually told that he did not look well.

The worst psychology in the world is the one that permits anyone to forget this fact and suggest to friends that they do not look well; for this is enough in too many cases to start a self-examination that does indicate something that can be construed as illness, with all the physical, mental and spiritual suffering that go with conditions less than health.

One need not go so far as to say that all illness is an idea, and that if the idea is corrected the supposed illness will disappear.

One must recognize the fact that the mind does react for good or ill on the body, and must realize not less that the body does react on the mind to exactly the same degree.

Thus the vicious cycle. The body imposes on the mind sensations that are not pleasant, suggestions of illness, and the mind becomes depressed accordingly. The depression of mind partially inhibits normal function, for all function depends on normal brain or nerve stimulus to act fully. So as the body depresses the mind, just so does the mind depress the body, the one making the other worse till actual illness or functional failure is the result, even in the end organic disease.

Joyful news peps us up, makes us forget physical handicaps, and actually improves health.

Depressing news does the reverse, depressing function, as it always does, and the vicious cycle is in full swing.

We can begin at either end of the cycle (if a cycle can be imagined to have an end) and break this chain.

If we can have such an uplifting psychology as to stimulate a normal physical function, then we have started improvement from the psychological aspect, while if we can set our physical house in better order we will have broken the vicious cycle from the physical aspect.

We can do both at once and produce still more rapidly effective results.

The physical is easily within our control if we adhere to the simple rules for nourishment already set forth. From the purely physical aspect with which the physician works, this is the logical point of attack, while the metaphysician would take the other view, and attack the vicious cycle from the psychological side.

In any case we must not lose sight of the mental influence on the physical, and the equal physical effect on the mental.

If you have had the privilege of knowing one of refreshing psychology, who never seemed or acted depressed, who was full of sunshine and good cheer, who spoke no evil of others, because believing no evil, who so thoroughly enjoyed life that all about him partook of this joy of living, then you have had one contact that should be cherished as long as life lasts, and you have witnessed the expression of a healthy physique.

If you have contacted the reverse of all these delightful attributes, forget such a person, and remember that such an one is not well.

Healthy function insures the former, abnormal function the latter; and the one who has "it," the one who attracts others as the flame attracts the moth, is well, full of ebullient health. We are always attracted by those qualities that we most admire, those qualities that we ourselves covet, while we are as surely repelled by the opposite qualities; thus it is not strange that the chronic ill lose their friends.

We see ourselves in others always, and can recognize in them the qualities we most portray, if we but see ourselves as others see us.

This is easily accounted for by the fact that we cannot understand qualities we do not ourselves possess to at least some degree. Thus the dishonest person trusts no one, the jealous one is as guilty of infidelity as the one suspected, else he would not be jealous.

And so, each friend is merely an outward portrayal of ourselves, so far as our appreciation of them is concerned.

We stimulate in others those qualities which are the most predominant in us, just as surely as a leaven leavens the whole.

If we wish to cultivate those qualities that we admire most in others then we can surely do this most effectively by making our bodies perfectly operating machines, as we can do through regenerating it in every part by a regenerative plan of recreation; for we are creating and recreating our physical parts continually; and the sort of body we have is under our full control, if we understand the law of replenishment.

Replenishment comes through replacement of the dying cells by the materials necessary for the recreation of these, and nothing else will do except exactly the materials necessary for their initial creation.

Nature provides all the materials necessary from the outgrowth of the soil of the earth, and we need nothing more.

We must have every one of the many elements necessary for this recreation of the body every day, and we must have these in form ready for use, combined with due respect to the immutable laws of chemistry.

If the body is unable in its present condition to keep itself fully cleared of its former debris of oxidation, then we must assist in such harmless ways as the enema, the purge, the sweat, exercise, sun baths, air baths, water bathing, till, as regeneration of tissue and function occurs, this assistance will be no longer required, and the regenerated body can again take care of its elimination of debris unassisted.

Thus the colon, crippled in function because of general body fatigue or functional decline, enervation, needs the assistance of the enema till its returning function makes this assistance unnecessary.

[189]

It may take five years to make a new body out of an old one, but suppose it required as many years as were represented by the degenerative changes present, even then it would pay enormously. But nature is very kind in this respect, for while the degenerative changes may have been going on for forty years previously, yet the complete regeneration may be accomplished in five years, or less, usually.

What if the changes through which the body must pass are not pleasant while the regeneration is progressing! We who have been through these realize that the day will break after awhile, just as it always does; and no matter how dark the night of change, the light of a returning vitality will surely break when we have unloaded enough of the deterrent debris to permit again of nearly normal function.

So, whether or not we understand the laws of psychology, we can at least set our internal physical realms in order, thus freeing the mind from impingement of deterrent physical sensations, and so prevent the vicious physical-mental cycle that is the road to disease in all its stages and phases.

When the body and mind are in harmony, only then will there be opportunity for proper spiritual development; for do not forget that the spiritual man is the first man, the mental the second, and the physical the third man; and only when these second and third are in harmony can there be a proper spiritual state.

Spirituality depends far more on a proper harmony of the rest of the man than is generally thought; and we have it in our power to create this harmony through proper understanding of the relationship of these two men, and the means necessary to keep them in harmony.

CHAPTER XVII.

Why a New Era?

ISN'T it about time for a new era in the understanding and the treatment of disease? When disease is rampant everywhere; when the health standard in our country is so low as at the present time, and degenerative diseases are continually on the increase; when our insane asylums are ever more crowded, our penal institutions overflowing; when the number of subnormal children is continually mounting, and the percentage of physical defectives in the average day school has equalled seventy-five per cent of the total enrollment; when after so many centuries of medical research and specialized and supposedly scientific treatment we are still confronted by such disheartening conditions in health; surely it is not unreasonable to predict and foresee a new era in the consideration of all the ills that afflict so great a percentage of our population.

The staggering total of surgical casualties is in itself enough to warn us that a new era must soon develop if we are to stop this decline in health and efficiency that is now the rule; and if we do nothing to change our conception of disease and the means for its control we will be compelled to admit that we are a second class nation or worse.

It is time for a new era in these matters. That it is in sight is the most hopeful sign of our troublous times. And it is in sight, as anyone can easily see who is in touch with the sick public continually.

A rather recent canvass of the residents of Chicago showed that but a small percentage of these were loyal to the medical treatment of their illnesses, the vast majority depending on the chiropractor, the osteopath, the Christian Scientist, the physiotherapist. Many had learned the sacred lesson of self-care and were dependent on no school or cult for the healing of the diseases that they have too well learned are self-created, and for which there is no remedy except self-care of the enlightened and understanding sort.

The writer for the past six years has been addressing groups in various sections of the country, sometimes very large audiences, and in every section there is this same reaction apparent, this turning away from the age-old medical idea and a seeking for light on this subject of self-care. It is often pathetic to see the eagerness with which they strive for a better understanding of the causes of many and varied illnesses that have for years made of their lives something scarcely to be enjoyed, often to be pitied.

After each lecture a period of at least equal length is devoted to the answering of questions; always these are to be written, and if signed the name of the inquirer is never revealed.

The almost monotonous burden of these is of the complete failure of medical treatment, often the recital of utter waste in treatment, every available dollar sacrificed in the search for health, and still no results; while in each case the whole history of physical failure is such a plain record of a progressive self-poisoning that it would seem too plain to be overlooked; and at every stage the habits producing the intoxication were correctible, if only someone had properly instructed the victim.

Too often the plaint is of what seems like needless neglect, or surely total indifference to the patient's own feelings and his own idea of the symptoms that were chiefly in evidence. Usually the patient has been treated as an infant without understanding, with no word as to the probable cause, no clear statement of the condition, and a seeming disregard for the patient's rights as the owner of the body under treatment.

Germany at the height of her paternalism was never quite like that. Verily, the medical machine is the acme of autocracy in its dealing with its devotees.

If you try to pin your doctor down as to the real nature of the troubles for which he has perhaps long treated you, he is too apt to feel that he is being cross-questioned, and to take offense at your evident lack of confidence in the infallibility of his judgment. You are almost sure to be treated to a dissertation in learned language liberally interspersed with Latin and Greek names and strange medical terms that leave you completely mystified. You may be greatly impressed with the great man's learning and the extreme complexity of your ailment, or you may be living in the new era to an extent, and realize that this man is merely using words to cover up his lack of exact knowledge.

If it is true, as often has been said, that "Words are given us to conceal our thoughts," then the average physician is usually successful, and he is following the advice of a learned teacher of medicine who always warned his students never to be too specific in telling patients of the nature of their troubles, as it might be too hard to take this back.

When as careful and scientific an institution as the Massachusetts General Hospital records forty-seven per cent of error in diagnosis, even after painstaking treatment and careful previous examination, as proved by their post-mortem findings, then surely there is not a great amount of exact knowledge of bodily conditions as they present for treatment.

It is not for a moment to be supposed that this institution is less exact than others, for its reputation is of the best, and its staff noted for their perspicacity and their conservatism.

Most institutions feel that they have fulfilled their extreme duty, justified themselves completely, when they have named the condition. If the naming is no more accurate generally than that admitted by this great hospital, then surely it is nothing that should justify the arrogance and unapproachableness of the usual type of physician when he attempts to tell his *patient* patient of the difficulties that in his august opinion are to blame for the present state of health or its opposite.

Surely the victim himself is entitled to as much consideration as is the employer in any line of construction work when he calls in a specialist in the line of work he is carrying on. The employer feels that he is entitled to the expert opinion he pays for, and with this the fullest personal understanding of the conditions present.

To autocratically announce to any ill person that he has developed a surgical condition and must at once lose some part of his anatomy of which he is perhaps very fond and that he thinks his very own, and without granting to this victim any right in opinion or desire, even without any attempt to enlist other opinion on the case, is to assume an attitude that is intolerable to any thinking man or woman, and one that will and should breed an attitude of passive or active resistance in those who have ever attempted to think for themselves.

It is this ignorance on the part of the sufferer in regard to his body and its function that opens the way for such infantile treatment; and it is extremely unfair for anyone to take advantage of this well known ignorance.

When any surgical operation is contemplated, other consultants, and chiefly of the internist persuasion, should be compelled by law. If all are agreed that operation is less dangerous than refraining from this *dernier ressort*, then let the subject be assured that the surgeon selected is competent and experienced, and make him post a bond sufficient to indemnify the victim, should the after condition be worse than the state preceding the operation. How much of the present surgery do you think would be performed? Not much. Perhaps less than the one per cent that the writer is willing to allow as possibly justifiable internal surgery, surely never more than this small percentage.

When Dr. J. F. Baldwin was retiring as president of the Ohio State Medical Society, he told them many truths, but his address was so plain and so uncomplimentary to medical methods that their journal refused to publish it.

Dr. Baldwin himself published it at his own expense, and it has been read and copied in part and republished in brief

[194]

form many times since, which was during the past ten or more years.

Dr. Baldwin was an old man at the time, perhaps well over seventy years of age, and generally recognized as the dean of the surgical profession in Columbus, even in the whole state.

He recited many of the well known surgical practices and condemned them, among others the reprehensible practice of fee-splitting. He did not hesitate to charge that the practice was all but universal among surgeons, which means that when your doctor calls in a surgeon he expects this surgeon to give him a third or more of the fee which you have paid him for his usually expensive operation, and you will see why this is so expensive.

Among other things he said that he had for years been taking his patients east to a certain large and noted clinic, and he had always been impressed by the fact that they had but two remedies, aside from surgery. One of these was nux vomica and the other was hope; but in the past few years he had observed a complete disappearance of nux vomica.

To name the condition is not constructive unless this leads to a constructive form of treatment; and surely internal surgery can never by any possible stretch of the imagination be called a constructive procedure, for it usually contemplates the removal of parts of the internal anatomy, and is a vandalism pure and simple, unless such removal is necessary to either prolong life or to ease intolerable suffering.

Surgeons do not like to hear such statements, naturally, and neither do they believe them, for they are trained in surgery. Surgery is their whole aim and object, and a successful operation is one that can be carried through to completion, whether or not the after condition of the subject of attack is improved.

A nice fat bond would do much to correct the tendency to unnecessary surgery, for not many surgeons would have the hardihood to assume any personal risk in performing any usual type of internal surgery, surely not so long as the patient can be persuaded to assume all the risks.

It is common practice today to request that the patient and his family sign a bond exempting the operator from prosecution should the operation fail, and this is in the nature of a waiver, no matter what the outcome of the operation, or even if the operator be found incompetent.

Nor is surgery greatly different from internal medicine in this respect; for while the internist does not require a waiver before administering any form of internal treatment, yet he is just as well protected against damage suits. No matter if his idea of proper remedies should cripple the subject, still he cannot be successfully prosecuted for the injuries sustained through his administration of remedies.

If the remedy used has ever before been employed in this or any other condition, or the dose prescribed be found in any medical work, then it is impossible to show the relation between the exhibition of the so-called remedy and the subsequent death or invalidism.

Of the many deaths resulting directly or indirectly from smallpox vaccination, or antirabic serum, or tetanus serum, or diphtheria antitoxin or toxin-antitoxin, or toxoid, or antistrepticoccic serum, or any of the host of other serums, not one has ever been brought home to the inquisitor who caused the death; nor can such be attached to him in any way, because these are legal forms of treatment, and the courts of law recognize only the orthodox authorities.

The writer is himself an Allopathic physician by education and can lay claim to no other school of education in medicine; yet he recognizes the practices of this school, his own school, as destructive always, and does not hesitate to charge this to his own profession, whether internal medicine or surgery is under consideration.

If a furnace man or a plumber wrecks your equipment you can have recourse to law to compel indemnification for your

[196]

loss; if a painter defaces your house through ignorance or incompetence, you would quickly seek damages; if an electrician bungles the wiring of your home so as to later cause fire, you would at once sue him for the damage caused, and you would probably win your suit.

But let a surgeon wreck your body, the most valuable machine of all, and you have no come-back; and do not forget that there are more surgical cripples today than those resulting from all other accidental happenings combined.

To lose the tonsils or the appendix is to place on the body a permanent handicap, not such as will terminate life, but such as will interfere with function in some or many ways so long as you live.

Constipation follows removal of the appendix as effect follows cause; also, the absence of tonsils opens the way for all sorts of infections later on, as witness the sore throats, the catarrhs, the sinus involvement, the frequent colds, bronchitis, following removal of the tonsils. Remember that nature creates nothing without purpose; and to remove any of the body organs is a vandalism against the future function of a body that should be conserved in all its parts and members if it is to continue to function as originally intended.

Because the hermetically sealed cavities of the body can be invaded without causing death is no reason for supposing that harm less than death has not been suffered by the victim.

Remember another thing, and that is that surgery cannot be done on your body without your consent; and do not let any surgeon frighten you into operation without first consulting several internists, men who are not sold to the surgical idea and have no profit visible from the performance of operations on your collection of organs that you call the body. To secure this consent the surgeon uses high pressure methods, of which fear is the chief weapon. Do not be frightened by some dismal surgeon, but seek other advice, and you will find to your

[197]

great surprise that opinions diverge so widely as to internal conditions that you come in time to feel that one man's guess is about as good as another's, perhaps better, and your own about as good as anyone's.

Fear kills indirectly by rushing one into needless danger through surgical mutilation; and it is unfair to use this weapon on those who do not understand.

Since the writer has definitely abandoned all surgical forms of treatment for internal conditions he has found occasion to refer but three cases to the operator during the past twenty-six years; and the cases that came under treatment were extremely often of the so-called surgical variety. Even in these three but one was found to be of such nature that the operative intervention could be called necessary.

One was merely an explanatory incision, on which the family insisted for business reasons, as it became necessary, they thought, for them to know whether the condition from which their father was suffering was cancer of the liver or cirrhosis; and this was one of those borderline cases in which there had been much disagreement. Incision showed it to be cancerous, and nothing could be done; so even this was useless except to satisfy the desire of the family.

The experience of this one observer would surely seem to indicate that the surgical necessities are not usually of the pressing variety, as the surgeon makes out.

Internal abscess, inflammations, infiltrations, adhesions, have disappeared with monotonous regularity when the whole man was subjected to radical detoxication and dietary correction.

If the surgeon could evaluate his results fairly, setting down in one column those results that actually improved the condition of the patient visibly, and in another column all adverse results, including deaths directly traceable to the operation, as well as all states that were not in any sense improved by the surgical work, he would indeed be a bold and bad man if he could continue to pursue his bloody calling.

The magnificent surgical clinics, with their polished tiles, their spotless cleanliness, their intriguing equipment, are very impressive. To have lived through a surgical experience is always considered a legitimate cause for congratulation, and people speak of these things and boast of them as of some great and heroic achievement.

"Speaking of operations," is the preliminary to many a painful recital of personal experience in such palaces of experiment.

It should be rather a sign of eminence to display no surgical scars on the entire body; but it would entail a paucity of conversation in groups that delight in these gruesome recitals, and who love to display their evidence.

We need a new deal, and we need it now and badly; but any lessening of surgical operations will not originate with the operators themselves, and scarcely will it originate with any part of the medical profession; for of all the monetary rewards in the practice of medicine, surgery is by far the most productive of any form of treatment, through fear of the calamities surgery predicts, as well as through the great reverence in which surgery is now held.

If your doctor tells you that you need an operation, do not permit him to call a surgeon to verify a surgical opinion, but insist on calling an internist, or two or three of these men who do not make their living out of surgery. If the opinion is still that operation is the only way out, then insist that the work be done by some competent man who has many successful operations to his credit, or one whose patients have not largely died as a result of his work. When such is selected insist that he post a bond to insure that he does not leave you worse than before; and make the size of the bond big enough to indemnify you at least in part for a life-long damage, perhaps semi-invalidism.

You will not find such a surgeon, of course, for anyone

who takes the lives of his patients in his hands daily without risk to himself is slow to see the fairness of this provision.

Yet you put any man under bond who is to handle your money, so why not the one who trifles with your life?

Better still, do not get yourself into such condition that any surgeon will have the opportunity to explore your interior; and you can do this, without doubt, if you follow all the suggestions before detailed for keeping the body up to par continually.

Eat less meats, eggs, fish, and cheese; eat the natural starches and sugars instead of the refined sort; take all your foods in compatible relation, the starches and sugars together with the vegetables, salads without acid dressing, sweet fruits or sweet desserts; take your proteins at a different meal, such as meats, eggs, fish, or cheese, and with these the vegetables, the salads, dressed with lemon juice and oil or cream, or with plain sour cream, and all the fresh fruits you desire of the acid variety, but omitting the starchy and sweet things; keep the colon up to date by daily use of the cool enema, as described before; keep up as much physical activity as possible without great fatigue; breathe plenty of good fresh air, drink only pure water, and do not avoid the sun.

These are all nature's remedies for failing health, nature's preventives for departures of all sorts from normal function or normal health. Only you can apply any one of them, so only you can keep the body right and so avoid the necessity of either surgical or medical treatment that may make your chances for comfortable old age something very problematic, if not extremely doubtful.

After all, you are your own keeper; and if you keep yourself well you need not worry about any form of treatment of any kind; and if you do not keep yourself so, the surgeon, the physician, the druggist, and even the mortician will become interested in you.

L'Envoy

FOR each of us there is some mission in life if we but
find it.

All have some definite thing to do, something for
which they have been created; and only the doing of this thing
will justify their existence here on earth.

If we come into the world and occupy space and time without giving anything back for this privilege, we have not justified ourselves, and our lives in the end are barren.

The humble writer of the foregoing work, modest as it is,
had from early boyhood a leaning toward the study of medicine, and never seriously considered any other field of usefulness; yet after thorough medical training and sixteen years of
medical and surgical practice, he knew that relief from disease
did not lie in the accepted channels of practice.

It required a personal breakdown and a hopeless outlook
for the future to really open his eyes to the possibilities of
relief from disease along entirely different lines, however un-
orthodox these at first seemed.

For twenty-six years he has abjured the usual methods and
has adhered to the so-called natural forms of treatment; and
each year of this practice has added to his firm belief that in
medical training we are wasting time needlessly, sacrificing opportunity for really constructive work, in a too close study of
pathology, or the science of disease, thus magnifying the abnormal at the expense of the normal.

This growing realization has so completely changed his
whole outlook on the subject of disease that it has become extremely difficult to listen patiently to organ recitals or the re-
tailing of endless symptoms; for he realizes plainly the incon-
sequential character of these.

He realizes that concentration on health and normal function instead of on the evidences of disease will almost at once improve disease states, for the more anything occupies the thought the larger does it become. With this realization it is easy to see that the more we think about disease the larger does the realization become, and, conversely, the more thoughts of health occupy the mind the more distinct does health-realization become.

If repetition in the foregoing work seems monotonous, please remember that any unusual and strange fact needs almost constant reiteration till it becomes an acceptable part of the daily thought, habitual thinking, almost.

The application of the principles before set forth, continued for twenty-six years on many thousands of almost every conceivable departure from health, has not only not weakened the first inspiration along these lines, but has actually every year deepened this into a fixed conviction; and the teaching of this doctrine has become a sacred mission.

The almost monotonous regularity with which diseased conditions of various kinds tend continually toward recovery, has taken away every fear of failure in applying these principles; and only lack of time or the unwillingness of the ill or their lack of co-operation defeats the ultimate recovery from disease and complete return to health.

If the assurances along these lines seem overplayed or exaggerated, remember that this is only by comparison with accepted standards of treatment, which have long taught the uncontrollable character of disease. To fully appreciate the conservative truthfulness of the attitude here taken one must experience at least a part of the results already long observed by the writer.

The continual enthusiasm of those who have through these simple means been led back from pain and discomfort and hampering disease to a state of real enjoyment of life is in itself sufficient warrant for the continuance of the methods advocated and continually employed by the writer and his associated staff.

The few thousands who have already benefited by resident treatment are but small in comparison to the thousands who have benefited through reading of the methods or studying and following the home course of management. The letters of thankfulness and appreciation received daily from so many who are complete strangers testify to the fact that the methods are so simple and effective that they can be successfully applied at any distance from personal supervision.

If the reader has been able to disassociate his thought from the prescribed conventions, and has accepted the doctrine of health creation through observance of simple rules that recognize laws long existing and long neglected, then he is in position to begin to apply personally the teaching of this unpretentious document; and he is also in position to realize early the reasonableness and truthfulness of the entire teaching. Such will have inaugurated a new era in health, and only so will the writer feel justified in setting forth what may be looked on in many quarters as unwarranted assumption.

Too often the errors of today were supposed to be the discoveries of yesterday, but only time and patient trial will show the truth or the error of any doctrine.

The surprising fact of entire self-control of disease is not at first easy to realize in the face of much erroneous medical teaching; but personal application of the principles as laid down in this work will convince the most skeptical of the demonstrable truth of the whole proposition. It is urged that each so modify his or her habit in the use of foods as to make this conform to the standards before laid out in this recital, and the writer is willing to be judged finally by the result.

We are entering a new era in the understanding and the

management of disease, and it would be well for everyone to realize this fact and set about adapting the daily life to the changed conditions, as otherwise a patient and sympathetic listener to symptom recitals may be difficult to find. May this time speedily arrive!

COMPLETE HOME PLAN

In his book, "A NEW HEALTH ERA," Dr. Hay has outlined thoroughly his principles and theories. To put these into actual practice at home, several helpful yet inexpensive items are published including a kitchen food chart, a leather-bound Pocket Guide, (both have complete food classification) a cook book with over 2000 compatible recipes arranged in menu form, and a monthly magazine with question and answer departments and menus for every day in the month.

(Those interested in reducing weight should obtain a copy of "WEIGHT CONTROL" by William Howard Hay, M.D.)

For Complete Details Write

POCONO HAY-VEN
MOUNT POCONO
PENNSYLVANIA

INDEX

[207]

INDEX

INDEX

[209]

INDEX

INDEX

INDEX

Printed in the USA
CPSIA information can be obtained
at www.ICGtesting.com
LVHW021620161123
764167LV00028B/199